TRUSTING
YOUR BODY

TRUSTING YOUR BODY

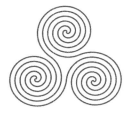

The Embodied Journey of Claiming Sacred Responsibility for Your Health & Well-Being

Susan McNamara

The Healer Within Series

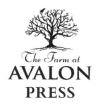

The Farm at
AVALON
PRESS

Paperback 978-1-958611-02-9
Ebook 978-1-958611-01-2

The Farm at Avalon Press
www.RememberingWhatMattersMost.com

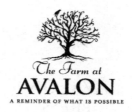

The Farm at
AVALON
A REMINDER OF WHAT IS POSSIBLE

To the body of the woman who gave me Life

To the bodies of my children that brought me back to Life

To the Body of the Good and Great Mother
that gives us all Life

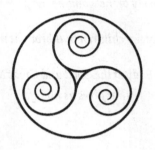

CONTENTS

Can you imagine a world of health and healing where each of us knew what was wrong with our bodies, how we got there and what we needed?

THE EMBODIMENT MANIFESTO

*A revolutionary commitment to
redefining how we care for ourselves*

Who we are and how we live matters

Honoring real human needs is fundamental to health

How we take care of ourselves
is our greatest contribution

Valuing our own life is valuing all Life

Personal health is a sacred responsibility

Self-care is built-in

Claiming bodily sovereignty is a
revolutionary act of health

Our bodies are Intelligent

Everything is connected

Good Medicine always begins with us

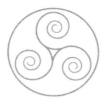

Journey Disclaimer

I imagine you're here because you're ready to begin *The Embodied Journey* of taking full responsibility for your body and your health. While predominant cultural norms tell you to outsource your authority and bodily sovereignty to experts, this view separates you from a vast and inborn Intelligence. To access this Intelligence, you must first learn to take full responsibility for your own body.

This is your body. It is yours to take care of. *This is non-negotiable.*

As you can see, this is not a legal disclaimer to avoid a lawsuit. This is so much deeper and more meaningful than that. I'm inviting you to make a necessary agreement with yourself to get very honest about the need to claim greater responsibility for the care and well-being of your own body.

Your health is literally in your own hands.

I'm not proposing you don't have healthcare practitioners you work with. And I am definitely not suggesting that you do not seek medical care when you need it.

What I am suggesting is that you develop the practice of consulting your own body first, before you look outside yourself for answers, treatments and cures. I'm suggesting that to be in a body responsibly, sacredly and authentically is a lifelong apprenticeship to the very Truth and essence of who you are and why you are here.

The Embodied Journey is a way of being that values connection and the preciousness of all Life. Beginning with your own.

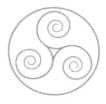

An Introduction to Your Body

"Just trust yourself, then you will know how to live."
- Johann Wolfgang von Goethe

You only get one body, and you will be with that body for the rest of your life. The relationship you have with your one body will be the most enduring one of your entire embodied existence. Does it not make sense then to cultivate a deep and trusting connection with this one body of yours? One that transcends doubts, self-loathing, fears, worries, distrust and agendas that undermine its healthy functioning, and your ability to feel good about being in a body.

You're being invited here into an awakening in how you look at this body of yours. How you treat it. How you feel about it. How you relate to it. The invitation being offered is to claim what is most necessary and natural in you when it comes to being in a body. So if you're open to the vast wisdom contained within you, along with the willingness to live like your body is yours to take care of, *you are in the right place*. This applies whether you are brand new at considering your body, or are more experienced in this way of thinking and being.

It can be easy to believe that our high rates of disease, illness and overall bodily disconnection are just the way it is now. But what if there is much, *much* more to this story? What if essential pieces have been left out when it comes to the basis of your health and well-being? And what if some of those missing pieces have to do with who it is that is actually responsible for your health, what your body truly needs and what it is that your symptoms are really all about?

Look around. There is an ever-growing awakening that we have strayed too far from what is good for us, and that expecting the technologies or other people to save us will only lead to further alienation from ourselves and the embodied intelligence available within us. Not to mention that we are not even getting the health results we desire. More to the point, our current mainstream medical approach seems to be incapable of saving us from the ill health and bodily disconnection that are far too common now, and that seem only to be accelerating; with greater levels of suffering on the rise now as we seek answers and quick fixes outside the realm of our very own embodied know-how.

This can be hard to hear. It can feel so much easier to believe that the fixes we seek for the body will be in a piece of machinery, an expert or a pill. That what these bodies of ours need most will come in the form of something far more intelligent than these bodies of ours. Something more infallible, orderly and guaranteed. Something safe because 'everyone' else is doing it, or because our doctor says so.

But what if this view is wrong? What if the reason so many of us are suffering so much in our bodies is because we have not started with what is real and true about who we are and what we most need? What if what we actually need is not complicated at all, but as simple and as close to us as our next breath? Or a well-placed question? Or a tending to one of our body's most basic and non-negotiable needs like hydration, real food, rest, movement or connection?

In a world that has normalized harming and mistrusting the body, *sometimes even requiring this as a way to fit in,* doing things differently from those around you requires great courage. We have such a powerful, survival-based need to belong that it can feel impossible to do anything but conform. To do what others are doing. To do what we are being told to do. No wonder it can feel so unsettling to trust these bodies of ours if it means doing things differently than those around us.

It's sad to say, but this describes the world we live in. One where we can no longer necessarily count on those around us to promote what is in our best bodily interests. We see this in the ways that we gather, making junk foods and screen time more important than health or being with the people we love. We see it in the rampant substance abuse that has become the 'new normal.' We see it in the fear-based and one-size-fits-all medical system that we 'must' rely on. And we see it in the barrage of pharmaceutical commercials always edging us towards subduing symptoms in the body as opposed to learning how to listen to them.

But how good is it for you, or the community for that matter, to continue to go along with what does not serve the very best in you? Or that even downright violates your body's most fundamental requirements and your trusting relationship to it.

If you're reading this, I imagine you're feeling and sensing that there is 'something else.' Perhaps you're yearning for a respectful and trusting relationship with your body. One that is based more in kindness and generosity, than in uncertainty, criticism or fear. Or you might be noticing that despite all the medical advances we have, too many of the guarantees we have been given *have not only failed*, they have created new problems all their own.

The 'something else' that many of us are feeling deep within, is what I think of as the call to *The Embodied Journey*. A natural movement towards who we really are through the exploration and the discovery of what a body needs. A commitment to honoring the sacred nature of our bodies and what they have to tell us. A way of living that says to you and everyone around you:

This life of mine is precious.

I deserve better.

We all deserve better.

This revolutionary call, and make no mistake about it, *it is indeed that*, bears many gifts. Ones like gaining greater respect for our own lives, feeling more confident in making life-affirming choices, finding our own voice in the midst of confusing and body-denying agendas and much, much more that only you can discover by answering this call. Ultimately, enabling you to know yourself as a trustworthy source of support and guidance for yourself when it comes to matters of life in a body.

What we're doing here may not look like anything you've been told, anything that gets advertised or anything that anyone thinks you should do when it comes to taking care of your body. Most of all, this journey may have nothing to do with what you've already tried, or where you believed healing would come from.

Instead, what I'm offering here is a new worldview on how to care for yourself, and it's for those of us who are open to that 'something else.' Those of us who are open to the idea that who you are and how you live matters, that your body is Intelligent, that symptoms are important, and even sacred messengers worth listening to, that your ability to care for yourself is built-in and that your health is ultimately in your hands.

What a big deal this all is! Such a big deal in fact that many of us shy away from taking this journey. Certainly we can look at all the ways we have been conditioned to not trust or believe in our bodies. And then there are all our experiences of past traumas, living in a body-commodifying culture, marketing gimmicks, being caught up in distractions and busyness that disconnect us from our bodies, and more.

But here's the good news. *Your body is always here.* Always responsive to your attention and efforts. Always available to serve as a portal into a deeper exploration of YOU. To what you need. To navigating our chaotic world with more clarity. To serving as a solid foundation for more satisfying relationships. To living with greater meaning and purpose. To knowing when something is off, despite what everyone around you is pulling for, or pressuring you to choose.

Best of all, *you don't need to have all the answers.* Or even much information. As a matter of fact, more information is not the solution. If that were true, the Information Age would have delivered all the health and wellbeing we could ever have asked for. That has not happened, and there is a good reason why.

There is a vast difference between being in and with your body and amassing advice and information about it.

What we need more of than anything else is to come back home to our own bodies, while learning how to listen to them from the inside-out. From the inside-out is exactly where our starting and ending point here together will be. Learning to be more in your body, while deeply and thoughtfully listening to its messages and guidance is the heart and soul of this journey. This does not mean it will always be easy or obvious. *It won't.* Being in a body is the ride of a lifetime. Sometimes thrilling. Sometimes terrifying. But it's the only way we get to be here. So why not make the most of it? Why not learn to listen in a new way? Why not support and cherish it to the very best of your ability?

How you live in and with your body matters. To wait for something to break down and get a replacement part or

just take pills and schedule procedures to make symptoms go away, while leaving it all in someone else's
hands, is to deny your very experience of being alive
and what your body is capable of.

It is to live distant from, afraid of or at war with, your
very own body. It is to suffer and to live separate from
every other form of life on the planet. It is to not know
who you are and what your place in the world is. It is to
act in the world from a disconnected, desperate and
destructive mindset. And it is to contribute to the creation of a world that works for no one.

Waking up to our own bodies wakes us up to everything
around us. But it takes time, patience, courage and
most of all, love, devotion and reverence to build that
level of connection with yourself. To be so intentional
about your relationship with your body that the natural
result is the knowing that you are valuable enough to be
cared for.

How to Use This Book

Everything contained here is offered as support and
encouragement to help you redefine how you care for
yourself. Everything is an invitation to see your body
with fresh eyes. While this will sometimes ask you to
challenge outdated beliefs or habits, never, *ever*, is anything said here a prescription, a pressure, a have-to or

a judgment. While at times the words may feel penetrating, it is always done in the spirit of helping you get unstuck in the service of greater connection to your body.

You are the ultimate authority on yourself. To that end, do what works for you. Make this journey your own. Go in any order of reading the chapters that you feel called to. If something doesn't fit or make sense, drop it. You might cycle back at another time. You might not. Take what resonates and leave the rest. Think of this as a kind of meandering around with your own body; akin to following breadcrumbs through the forest. Allow yourself to be guided and to be led from one thing to the next without a preconceived idea about how you have to go.

If you want to skip around, here's how I've imagined what you have in your hands. The very core of you being able to trust your body is distilled down in the chapters, *You Must Be in Your Body, You Must Be Willing to Learn the Language of Your Body* and *You Must Be Willing to Break From a Sick Herd*. Together, these three give you the foundation you need to reclaim sacred responsibility for your health and well-being.

The chapters, *Body Basics* and *Obstacles* expand on and support this foundation, with *Getting Your Bearings* serving as the set up to get you started. You might want to begin here as this chapter is a body of teachings unto itself, and something you could work on for the rest of your life. But again, wander around wherever you feel most called.

And if you only have a moment, go to any of the experiential sections outlined in gray to take you right into the experience of your body. *This is the most important place to go, always. For there is a vast difference between reading about your body, and being in your body.* The experiential sections will help you get to the latter, faster.

However you take this journey, the only litmus test you might want to use as you go through these pages is: *Does this bring me closer to trusting my body or further away?*

We will both have done our jobs well if when you read certain parts, you have the experience of *"I knew that!"* The Embodied Journey is an experiential one. As in, you must be willing to be in your body and be with what is there. So even if you currently feel disconnected and removed from your body, your capacity to inhabit it fully, lives on within you and seeks only for you to connect back in.

So include it all. Even the stuff you don't want.

Finally, it's essential that you practice what you find here. Or some version of it. *Daily*. You cannot just read something and expect that your body, or your relationship to it, will magically change. To be in a body in a healthy and satisfying way is to ultimately go beyond information, your fears and hang-ups, other people's ideas and cultural norms. That takes practice. *Lots of it.*

So take the experiential suggestions, try them on and make them your own. If you can do this, the practices will become habits, which will become ways of being, which will then go on to create a more trusting relationship with this one body of yours.

A Few Last Things

- **We all have good reasons for resisting and distancing ourselves from our very own bodies.** Some of those reasons are protective, some are habitual and some are encouraged by the culture. It's not always easy to know or experience things about ourselves. Especially if we haven't been paying attention to our bodies and what they need. For many of us, what we initially resist may be one of the richest places to explore because it can reveal our habits, conditioning, taboos and unconscious beliefs. *If we are willing to see it that way.*

- **This brings us to trauma.** We all have it to varying degrees. It's near to impossible to not have experienced trauma in the times we live in. While I am someone very attuned to personal and collective traumas *this is not a book about trauma.* The focus of this book is on what is possible when we learn to make our way back into our bodies in a natural, loving and healing way. You know yourself best. If this is not for you, don't do it. If things come up, get the help you need. A big part of healing from trauma is not doing to ourselves what was done to us. *As adults, that choice is always in our hands.*

- **What you have in your hands is a primer.** While the book is not sparse in pages (how could it be given the vast nature of the topic?), the spirit of the writing is that of a primer. Meaning, we are addressing the basics. The rest is up to you. So while I have tried to distill it down as best as I can, there is much that is not included here. Much that I may have not gotten just right for you. Don't let that deter you. Instead, use it to motivate you to explore. If something here doesn't work or is not complete for you, create it for yourself. Whatever you do, make it your own, while giving yourself a balanced blend of the time you need while simultaneously holding yourself accountable.

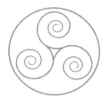

Getting Your Bearings

"You have set sail on another ocean, without star or compass, going where the argument leads, shattering the certainties of centuries."

- Janet Kalven

As you set out on The Embodied Journey of learning how to claim sacred responsibility for your health and well-being, *you need support.* You need ways to understand what it means and what it takes to trust your body in the midst of navigating the potentially new and uncharted waters of living your embodiment with more intention and greater connection.

I often think of us going from our current (and often outdated) models of the body, health and what is possible, as the equivalent of going from *the earth is flat to the earth is round.* It took hundreds of years for that shift to occur, with lots of bumps and resistance along the way. But for those of us who embraced this radical truth early on, what an amazing world of possibilities it opened up!

It is no different with the body.

When it comes to trusting your body, getting your bearings means figuring out where you are so that you can decide what is most true about your body, what you most need and how to get to where you most want to be. This is less about a destination, *and more about a life-long journey*. One that we must all take, one way or another. Why not go with a compass and map in hand? Why not accept the unknowns of this journey in the spirit of greater health and self-awareness?

Why not learn how to be in your body, caring for it, and honoring it in a respectful and sacred way?

What follows are six navigational points on The Embodied Journey map to help you explore life in a body without getting sidetracked by fear, disconnection or doubt. Think of this chapter as support mixed with sustenance to help you make the trip. Use the points as you would markers on a map to help orient and anchor you whenever you feel lost. Most of all, enjoy the trip!

One final thought before we get into the specifics. While it can be natural to feel overwhelmed at times by the vast ocean that is your body, *don't let that stop you.*

Even a small thimble holding a tiny amount of ocean water possesses all the qualities of the ocean. *Is in fact, the ocean itself.* What this means is, each time you learn even a little bit more about this vast and mysterious body of yours, you come to know yourself beyond diets, self-loathing, someone else's opinion, fears and more. Every single part of your journey is valuable and ultimately serves as the very foundation of you trusting yourself.

That's precisely how it all started for me. When I was in my mid-twenties, after years of trying different diets, I made a commitment to stop attacking myself over this thing called being overweight. *My first act?* Getting rid of the judge and jury I submitted to every single morning. Better known as the bathroom scale. My second act was to begin the lifelong process of taking a closer look at why I was using food to stuff down emotions and beat myself up with.

I never set out to do anything in particular, or in any particular order. As a matter of fact, my first adventure came in the form of being sick and tired of yo-yo dieting and the self-hatred that went with it. Exhausted with using a number to tell me whether I was good or bad, I was finally ready to try another way. *Though I literally had no idea what that way was.*

I didn't know what the journey would ask of me, where I would wind up *or even if I could do it*. The only thing I knew was that I was ready for something else, and that I was going to approach my life on my terms. Which meant it wasn't going to look like what I was being told I needed to do to get control of my body. Decades later, what I can tell you is this: It wasn't about measuring up to some external, *or even internal*, standard. It wasn't about getting something, or becoming something that I wasn't already. And it definitely wasn't about someone else's version of what I should do.

Instead, it was about remembering what my body already knew. My ability to care for myself and know what I needed came with me at birth. It was hard-wired in and nobody else's business to tell me how to do it or what it should look like. Has it ever been derailed? *Yes.* Forgotten? *Absolutely.* Misled? *For sure.* Lost for good? *Never.*

Now you.

---

1. Begin Where You Are

BEING IN YOUR BODY

Beginning where you are is the ultimate embodied homecoming. To get there requires accepting what your body is experiencing at any given moment. *Even when you don't like what's there.* As hard as this can be, there's no way around this one. If you hope to live in a body you feel good in and can trust, you must be willing to actually *be in it.*

This might sound ludicrous, as in, *where else would I be?* That's the trouble with being human. We can be anywhere but in the body when the mind takes us into the past or the future. The past keeping us locked in old fears, traumas and beliefs. The future serving as a source of great anxiety and uncertainty on the one hand, and on the other hand, as the fantasized place where everything will somehow be magically better down the road.

When the mind automatically goes into the past or the future, we have left our bodies without the fully present mind that it needs to be whole, clear, balanced, grounded and secure. And a mind not in the present moment will generate thoughts and habits that have nothing to do with where our body is or what it needs.

To begin where you are is to accept your body exactly as you find it.

I mean this literally. You must be willing to locate yourself just where you are in the nuts and bolts and nitty-gritty of life in a body. You must acknowledge what you find there including all of the thoughts, the emotions, the pains, the sensations, the urges, the instincts and the intuitions contained within you.

This is no different than mapping out a road trip. If you don't know where you're starting from, *if you aren't in the vehicle to begin with*, how can you possibly reach your destination? How will you know what it takes to make the trip? How will you know if you've taken a wrong turn? Being in your body means being with what you typically try to get away from, and while just the thought of this may have you ready to bolt, *stay with it.*

ACCEPTING THE SHIFTING STATES OF YOUR BODY

We want our bodies to be the same, forever and ever. We see this in the culture's obsession with youth. The name of the clothing store, *Forever 21* says it all. As do the tech filters we use to make us look younger. Not to mention all the creams, the whiteners and the procedures to shave off the years or make us look thinner.

But the truth is, healthy bodies simply do not, and cannot, stay the same forever and ever. Yet many of us continue to hold some belief that there's a perfect state to cling to or try to get back to. Maybe it's a vision of yourself at the age of sixteen. Or that summer when you were twenty-two and had successfully starved yourself into the smallest size you've ever been. Maybe you carry an image of yourself that's never even existed, wishing to look like some celebrity that you admire.

To be in a body that honors who you are is to acknowledge that your body is different year to year and day to day. *Even moment to moment.* This means that unfamiliar, uncomfortable and unwanted changes, according to the conditioned mind and the culture at large, must be accepted. *Even honored.*

But in a world fixated on certainty and uniformity, our body's changing ways do not always sit well with us. So while it's only natural to want the body to always feel and look good, that's just not realistic. More than that, it puts us at odds with ourselves and our shifting states as we fight against what is.

Some days the body is going to hurt, *and it may never measure up to some idealized standard.* At times we will be afraid, confused or ashamed by what is there. But if we refuse these experiences, our attempts to distance ourselves from what we don't want or like will result in us becoming disconnected *from our very selves.* And by extension, Life itself.

Honoring the body means accepting variability, change, differences, unknowns and yes, *even discomfort.* Perhaps hardest of all, you must accept the changing image in the mirror without pulling away or using it as a daily opportunity to criticize yourself.

SUSPENDING JUDGMENT IS A MUST

To begin where we are also means no more judging the body. No good. No bad. No right. No wrong. Not with others. Not with yourself. This goes for all those comments that pop up in your mind whenever you see your own reflection. It also goes for the fantasized versions of yourself as told to you by the spell casters (aka the marketing firms) or by disingenuous social media posts you know are BS but that you hand your power over to just the same. Comparing yourself to what is not real or to an unfair assessment of yourself, while obsessing about how others have it better or more figured out than you do, is a recipe for a deep distrust and loathing of your own body.

But maybe you believe that being critical of your body is an effective way to motivate yourself or even, to fit in. Maybe you're thinking, *If I don't judge and compare myself against some external standard to determine how I'm doing, won't all of my vices and laziness run the show?* No.

Judging is nothing more than banishing your body, while undermining and devaluing your very existence; your very right to be alive in an easeful and joyous way coming under attack in the shadow of judgment. As in, if our body parts don't measure up, we are somehow less than. Not just in our eyes, but in the eyes of the world as well. Judgment makes the challenges of the human experience much more painful than it needs to be. While we will not always be able to control what the body is doing, *we can absolutely change how we relate to it.*

WALKING THE UNKNOWN PATH

Walking the unknown path means welcoming in the unfamiliar in life. On The Embodied Journey, you will absolutely encounter territory you have not explored before. It's more than okay that you don't know where you are or which direction to go in. What matters most is that you let yourself be where you are, while suspending judgment that you should know better than you do.

On the unknown path, it's essential to learn how to be a good travel partner to yourself. While it's easy to get down on yourself when you're lost, it's far wiser to be good to yourself as you go. Truly, you are no better or worse off if you're starting your journey in the south as opposed to the north, or in the night as opposed to the day. There are no awards to be won, or penalties to be assessed because it takes you more or less time than anyone else, because you went a different way, got lost and needed help, or that it looks really messy and unfinished to yourself or others.

This is the journey of more than a thousand steps that begins with you taking one step at a time, while allowing the experiences your body is having to guide you. This includes taking in as many of the sights, smells and sounds as you can. Knowing that as you head off into the unknowns of your very own body, there will be voices, both yours and others, that will tell you, *don't do it, you won't make it, you'll fall off the edge or be eaten by sea monsters.*

Two things:

1. This is to be expected.
2. Don't believe them.

2. Your Body is Your Responsibility

CLAIMING SOVEREIGNTY

It is a massive developmental leap to go from outsourcing your sovereignty to claiming it.

By sovereignty I mean one who is self-determined, free and independent. A sovereign being is "an acknowledged leader" according to the dictionary. This is you being the leader of your own body by claiming full responsibility for it. In other words, *The Embodied Journey is one of going from being a child who looks to others to tell them what to do, to the grownup who claims agency over their own life.*

Claiming authority in this way is the very foundation of embodied self-trust. For until you can embrace that what goes on with your body is up to you, you will fall into the trap of outsourcing your wisdom and personal power; trading it for a false sense of security and safety as promised to you by another. While it may feel like a surer bet to leave your body in the hands of another, this belief robs you of full status. And when adults continue to live like children instead of fully sovereign, it robs the world of seasoned elders to keep wisdom and experienced perspective alive to pass down to the generations to come.

As an adult, leaving your bodily decisions in the hands of another is a dicey choice, even when that outside person has your best interests in mind. In worse case scenarios, you may be leaving your body in the hands of someone who is only interested in furthering their own agenda. This can take the form of the billion-dollar diet industry, the profit-driven medical industrialized complex, a social media influencer or a pharmaceutical marketing campaign. *Taking responsibility for your body relates to EVERYTHING you do in life and is a process that unfolds over time.*

Well, you might say, *I'm no expert.* That's what the doctors and other professionals are for. They're the ones in charge of what happens with my body. After all, they know best. *Who am I to know what my body needs? Who you are is the only one in the whole wide world who will ever know what it is to live in your body!* You are the only one who knows what it feels like to be you and who can hear the unique messaging of your own body. Only you know how to respond in exactly the right way.

I know this place intimately through my initiation into motherhood and beyond. I walked this part of the journey when I was deciding what to do when it came to the bodies of my children. Hands down, this was one of the most difficult *and* affirming things I have ever done in my life.

Because my husband and I made choices around our kids' bodies that fell outside of mainstream medicine, mass media marketing and what the culture in general was offering, I was confronted *daily* with having to choose whether I would go along with those expectations or choose what made the most sense to me about what I thought a body truly needed to thrive.

Nothing before or since has grown the deep sense of core responsibility I take for my own life, like choosing for the bodies of my children. It all felt like such high stakes at the time. And yet, it was exactly that feeling that pushed me to get clearer than ever about whose job it was to claim responsibility for my life and what I was choosing. The experience of motherhood has forced me to own the choices I make; separate from my fears, the responses from others, my past and any pushback from the conventional medical system.

When I first began, I had no idea what I was being schooled in. Looking back now, I recognize that all of the challenges, all the times I chose differently, all the tears and loneliness, the doubts and the frustration, were teaching me how to think for myself. How to choose for myself. How to be my own person. How to be the healthiest and most autonomous version of myself, while still belonging to those around me.

I cannot say exactly what it will be for you when it comes to the lessons and the gifts available as you take responsibility for your body. I can only say that you will not be the same and that from that lack of sameness will arise a most unique and amazing individual who will serve as a blessing to not only themselves, *but to all of us.*

DEVELOPING TRUSTED PARTNERSHIPS

Does claiming responsibility for your own body mean you go it alone? *Absolutely not.* It is essential that you have a circle of practitioners, friends and community you trust and who respect your voice when it comes to your health. Life (health being a huge part of that) is after all, a co-creation. We have always relied on collaborations with others around our bodies where wise counsel and support based in integrity are an integral part of making solid choices.

At its best, our health partnerships are with those we can create a sacred trust with; collaborations that generate far more wisdom and insight than we might discover on our own. These partnerships offer us the kind of support that brings out the very best in us, that lifts us when we are low and that reflects back to us what we are truly capable of. These are healing relationships that allow you to factor in all that you need, and that support you in filtering all of it through your beliefs, faith, goals, intuition and aspirations, *along with your very own body and what it needs*, when deciding how you need to best proceed.

Never are you bullied, coerced or shamed. *Never* are you told you don't know what you're talking about or that what you're experiencing is insignificant. *Never* does an insurance code dictate your care. *Never* does someone limit what is possible in your body. *Never* do you allow yourself to be treated like a child. These are just some of the deep and powerful personal stands you must make in order to claim sacred responsibility for your own body. While not quick or easy, I know it is possible for you, because this is precisely what happened for me.

Right about now, you might be thinking, *how can I do this?* Given our current understanding of what healthcare is, it might seem impossible to find a practitioner who would value your insights. I encourage you to begin to expand your understanding of what health and healing is to consider a wider interpretation of what this might look like for you.

Perhaps there is a role model in your life, someone you see as vibrant and alive that you could spend time learning from. Or maybe there are healing modalities you have heard about that you could research. Or perhaps you have a friend or co-worker who has had great success with an approach you never heard of before. You could also be on the lookout for communities building a new approach to how we care for ourselves. It's a new concept but I know they are out there because this is something I am in the process of exploring and creating with others through my own health and healing community called *The Healer Within*.

I know it can feel like a lot to do in the beginning. Equally though, it is an incredibly empowering journey to dig this deep into what you truly need. This is an absolute prerequisite to you developing self-trust. The journey of embodied co-creation you take with others is filled with enormous possibility when you can find guides who help you come home to your own body, while supporting you in taking full responsibility for what is yours to do.

THERE ARE NO GUARANTEES

Every human being wishes for a guarantee for how our lives will turn out, especially when it comes to health and the body. It seems so much more palatable to believe that if we put our bodies in someone else's hands, we'll get the results we want, minus the need to make difficult choices. That by leaving it up to someone else we can bypass the uncertainties of life in a body. Only... *it's not true.* Life in a body comes with no guarantees. No matter whose hands we put it in. Our own included.

You cannot be in a body in any kind of real and satisfying way without accepting this. You cannot sidestep this reality by having someone else tell you what to do. You cannot secure something by doing what everyone else is doing. To be fully responsible for your own body is not something that just happens to you or is done for you by someone else. It is something you must claim with eyes wide open to all of the realities of your existence. What you have control over. *And what you have absolutely no control over.*

This takes going beyond the bounds of your own fears, conditioning and insecurities to cross the unknown sea of yourself and your body. But by embracing the uncertainty and the 'no-guarantee clause' of living is precisely what will bring you great growth, clarity and empowerment. All vital qualities for a life well-lived in this body of yours.

3. Self-Care is Built-In

IT'S WIRED INTO US

At its most basic and most authentic, the capacity to care for ourselves is built-in. Hardwired into the nervous system. Into every cell, organ and tissue layer of a body that wants to live, *and live well*. This is a holy inheritance from all of the Intelligence of all of the Life that has ever come before you.

True self-care is native to who you are and does not require anyone else's permission. Nor does it require glitzy accouterments. As a matter of fact, real self-care is not fancy or only for those with disposable income. You are gifted with an inner-knowing of body-based self-care. It is bestowed upon you as a birthright. It is there in the matter-of-fact rhythm of your daily life and it cannot be reduced down to massages, manicures or splurges. That mentality is an insult to its true power and rightful place in your life.

I propose you think of self-care as a way of attending to, honoring and protecting your truest nature. Wow! How might that change things for us to be working at that level?

Right about now, you might be thinking: *Are you kidding me? That sounds like a lot of work to get to know myself at that level!* True. But what I know is this: Being unable to care for or trust your own body is far more work than what it takes to get to know yourself. Not having the energy or stamina to enjoy your life and do the things you want to do is a far more difficult and burdensome existence than exploring what's already in you. Feeling hatred, disgust or mistrust towards your own body causes more suffering than any effort you might make to care for it by a longshot.

You might also be thinking, *where's the proof?* How do you know self-care is built in? The answer is mirrored in nature; we're mammals after all. No mammal can survive if it doesn't know how to take care of itself. Sadly, this is exactly where we're at as a species. We have become so separated from the innate know-how around how to care for ourselves, that with each passing generation, we grow increasingly sicker. *On every single level of human life.* Despite all of the information, technologies, hospital mergers, healthcare, insurance, specialists, smoothies and more, we have never been more ill, out of shape and confused about what is happening in our very own bodies.

Beyond looking for proof, what would be possible if we embraced the paradigm that we did, in fact, know how to take care of ourselves? Even if we've strayed. Even if we never got a good example growing up. Even if the environments we live in no longer reflect or support that. *What might be possible for all of us to embrace that our self-care is a built-in birthright?*

IT CANNOT BE LOST TO YOU

Finally, because your ability to care for yourself is hard-wired into you as a mammal, *it can never be lost to you and it goes with you wherever you go.* How could it be any other way? Without the ability to care for yourself, you could not survive. Never mind thrive.

So even if right at this moment you don't feel connected to your built-in capacity of inner self-care wisdom, even if you feel like you've lost it, or maybe never had it to begin with, it does not mean that it is not there. It only means that you need to turn towards it. You do this one day at a time, and it is precisely this 'turning towards' that will develop the precious connection to what is wired into you, and that can guide you as you make your decisions when it comes to your body

Your innate capacity to care for yourself wants nothing more than to be expressed, fully and completely. And if you are not feeling connected to this right now, just know that what we are doing here together is part of a larger process of bodily reclamation that includes you, and that is more than you. In other words, you're not alone, and you're on the right track. No matter where you're starting from.

4. Everything is Connected

EVERYTHING INFLUENCES EVERYTHING ELSE

How we live, think, emote and relate all create and reflect what it feels like to be in a body. Everything going on in our personal and collective world makes its own unique imprint on us. In other words, *everything influences everything else.*

How you live, and what is happening around you, shows up in your body. What you eat, where and with whom you hang out, how many prescriptions you take, how you move and what you watch on a screen all contribute to the current and future state of your body. Whether you sit on a couch or spend time outside, believe in yourself or not, talk well of others or gossip, hold grudges or forgive, take your share or deprive yourself, *all of it* will find a place in your life, as expressed through your body.

Your feelings, your habitual responses, your connection to Source and to the natural world, who you admire, how often you live in fear or joy, how safe it feels to be you, how you feel about your childhood, the quality of the air you breathe and the soil you walk in and eat from, what is happening in your family and on the main stage of the world, all coalesce to create how you feel about the life you are living in the body you were given. All of it together is creating your health, *or lack thereof.*

Despite what we have been told, or how we have come to live, everything is influencing everything else. Nothing is separate from anything else when it comes to life in a body.

SEPARATION HARMS

The Western medical perspective *does not* see everything as being connected. Viewing a human body from a perspective of connection and wholeness, challenges a system that likes everything to be neat, orderly, linear and manageable. Accepting the truth of our body's wonderfully holistic nature has far too many variables for a system that demands efficiency, eschews outliers and belittles the unknown.

Our conventional medical system focuses on fixing and replacing broken parts when it comes to our bodies. Just like we would with a machine. Just like the machines being used to treat us now. Things like emotions, our past, big systemic failures, pollution or our lack of connection to meaning and purpose are viewed as too messy, too contrary to insurance codes, too time consuming to the twelve-minute office visit, too outside the purview of medicine and definitely, too 'unscientific.'

In our conventional approach to medicine, each part of the body has its own specialist now. We treat one part as if it were an island unto itself. A physician might prescribe medications to address something in the heart, only for this 'fix' to create problems in other organ systems. Now, a second pill is prescribed to counteract the side effects. This next drug creates another problem that must be corrected. On and on it goes, treating symptoms without getting to the root cause of the issue. Without asking deeper questions, or god forbid, connecting the seemingly disparate and inconveniently placed dots of everything that influences a person's body.

I saw this as my mother lay dying in the hospital under the care of no less than seven doctors. Not only was there little to no communication among them, *there was barely any interaction with her.* One specialist even proclaimed his stamp of good health on her *without him ever having been in the same room with her.* How had he come to his conclusion? Test results that told him that as far as his area of discipline was concerned, she was doing great!

And yet, there she lay, alternating between a nonverbal and fetal-like existence with wild-eyed and desperate attempts to communicate what she could not. Test results, oxygen saturation rates and their inability to find anything wrong notwithstanding, here was a woman who only a week prior had been alert, cognitively sound, living on her own and communicative.

It was maddening to watch them be unwilling to admit they had no idea what was going on as they subjected her to test after test after test. Infuriating to watch her be reduced to results on a screen. Disheartening to see the lack of recognition that an actual human being was in that bed. If I could do it all over again, I would have kidnapped her from the hospital, brought her home and crawled into bed with her. Which is where I began with her at the start of her hospital stay, but which became impossible as the days wore on with each new technological device brought into the room. Literally blocking me from getting physically close to her.

Nothing is separate from anything else when it comes to the body. Everything is touching and influencing everything else. To fully honor the truth of a human body is to not only recognize this, *but to be in awe of this.* It is to be guided and humbled by this. Everything in the body is aware of everything else in the body with a continual and ongoing communication occurring that defies the understanding of a modern mind that wants to separate it for convenience and easy understanding.

Does not the blood flowing through the body sense the condition of the organs through which it passes? Does a human body not register a lifetime of stress or trauma? Do we not see that the places human beings dwell impact them? Do we not recognize that the family a child is raised in impacts their whole life?

**Everything a human body comes
in contact with, inside or outside of itself,
is felt and known by that very same body.**

WE ARE MADE OF SOMETHING MORE

We are the very Intelligence that created the cosmos. There is Something far greater than us, is us, brings us here and enlivens the very nature of these bodies of ours. Call it what you will, but by whatever name you use, it is beyond the rationalities of the mind and it is being obscured in a world that has come to believe that human endeavors are the most intelligent force of all.

We assume the human mind is the greatest of all the forces in the Universe. That our human creations are superior, and that it is we who control Life itself; believing we can bend it to our will and do with it as we see fit. Nowhere is this attitude more prevalent than with our bodies. We mistreat them for years and then go to pills, procedures and the technology du jour to fix what we have broken. We act as if our bodies are machines, and that it doesn't matter how hard we are on them because the inventions of man will make up for our abuses. We believe that through the push of a button, we can alter whatever we have done to ourselves. And that if we only wait long enough, the next technological invention we come up with will clean up the mess we have made of ourselves and the world.

Because we can want something, click a button and get what we want, we have taken that same mentality into health. *At great peril.* That peril being the disconnect that arises out of the hubris of the rational mind that puts us above the Laws of Nature, the very ones that are meant to guide us in the world. Laws like the cyclical nature of Life which reveals that things come into existence, stay for a while and then leave. This natural rhythm shows us there is no reason to cling to one part of the cycle. No reason to expect the body to stay the same forever and ever.

Something More is always informing us. Always there. If we can only see it that way. Without recognizing that there is a Source in the world that is both more than us, *while also being us*, we will be forever disconnected from a higher understanding of what it means to live in these bodies of ours. What it is that we can appeal to, reference and use as a guide to keep us close to the Truth of who and what we are. Without which we run the risk of human arrogance with all of its blind spots and proclivity to harm through ignorance, separation and a grandiose and misplaced sense of its own limited power.

To live fully in the knowing that there is Something More than us is to take our rightful place in the order of things. It is to know our true power. Perhaps most of all, it is to know our own limitations, and then use that knowing as a necessary stopgap from creating a level of destruction that not only brings ill health and unhappiness to each of us, *but to the rest of the world as well.*

5. Your Body is Wise, Unique & Trustworthy

YOUR BODY KNOWS HOW TO HEAL

Your body is Intelligent and it knows how to heal. Every day your heart beats and pumps blood without you needing to remind it what to do. Your kidneys filter out what you no longer need and release it through your urine several times a day. When you cut yourself, your blood begins clotting without you needing to remind the body to activate its built-in first-aid response. An egg and a sperm come together and begin the miraculous process of creating a human being without us needing to orchestrate a single thing.

Because we have come to distrust the body, because so many of us now are so sick (without recognizing the hand we've played in this) we have come to believe that the body makes lots of mistakes and therefore, *cannot be trusted*. Our general sense is that these bodies of ours have gone haywire, so we need lots of outside help and complicated treatments to get them under control. That the body is inherently and fundamentally flawed, and therefore requires our vigilance, is unfortunately the common narrative we have taken up.

But what if the so-called mistakes we believe our bodies are making, *are not mistakes at all?* What if they are signals trying to get our attention, alerting us to how far we have drifted from what we most need? *What if what is really being called for is to trust that your body has very good reasons for whatever it's doing, and that it would be wise for you to figure out what that is?*

BIO-INDIVIDUALITY: YOUR UNIQUE NATURE

Along with the wisdom inherent in your body, you are also a unique individual unto yourself with a unique history and unique needs. So while human bodies have much in common, *you have your own version to get to know.* You are, after all, encoded with your own bio-individual imprint, life experiences, reasons for being here, along with particular challenges, gifts, goals, needs and sensibilities.

This is precisely why a one-size-fits-all medicine approach will never suffice. Unfortunately, we live in a world that worships at the altar of the assembly line approach to health. Hierarchical and top-down systems abound where some 'authority' at the top, usually a male, is in charge of those at the bottom. Our current system is imposed upon us (note how often you cannot opt out of the system for other types of care), is fragmented in its approach and owes its allegiance to an anonymous for-profit system more interested in the bottom-line than in treating us as unique individuals.

The experience I described with my mother in the hospital reflects this kind of approach. She, and her unique bodily experience, was not at the center of the equation of her care. Instead, the hospital codes and its protocols were. The forms, the insurance payouts and the doctor's rotation schedules were. None of this had anything to do with her, and what her body most needed.

This approach to the body gives orders, proclaims that things must be a certain way and that the patient must fit into the system as opposed to the other way around. It excludes and it does things *to* the body, not *for* or *with* the body. And it absolutely refuses to see that there is a unique human being with unique needs needing to be tended to.

That is the nature of the one-size-fits-all approach with its main aim being to keep the system running in an 'orderly' fashion. As a culture, we are so steeped in the robotic, automated, assembly line, hierarchical approach to the body that to contemplate that our bodies are uniquely intelligent and trustworthy can feel like too big of a leap to make. *Dangerous even.* As in don't you dare express a need that falls outside of what this system has deemed worthy of its time and effort. To do so is to risk condemnation. Maybe even a rejection of you from a doctor's office or insurance policy; a turning away from you when you are most in need because you don't fit the system's protocols.

You will know of what I speak if you or someone you know has ever questioned a doctor or some aspect of the medical system, only to be denied, demeaned, kicked out or ridiculed. Only to be told they will not treat you unless...*you comply with their version of you.*

On the other hand, a bottom-up approach is an organic and grass roots way of being that includes. *Everything.* Our uniqueness, the understanding of ourselves, our fears and limitations, what we need and what we can and cannot do. Bottom-up is a 'being with' that honors the individual, while meeting and greeting all the unique aspects of who we are as one coherent, unique and sacred whole.

This kind of approach is worth knowing and fighting for. A system of care and understanding about the body that banishes nothing. One that sees our totality, while embracing what it is that makes us uniquely who we are.

6. Learning to Be in Your Body is a Lifelong Apprenticeship

A NECESSARY DEVOTION

Your relationship with your body, and make no mistake about it, *it is a relationship*, is your most important one. Funny how little time and energy so many of us give to our most important and lifelong relationship. Maybe it's because we take it for granted, until of course it hurts or doesn't work. Or maybe it was so thoroughly shamed, ignored or denigrated while we were growing up, that it can feel too painful to be with it.

The repair to the rupture in this relationship cannot be rushed, forced or ignored. The body has its own timing that has nothing to do with the edicts of the rational mind, the latest hack or the time frames of the twelve-minute office visit. It has its own form of Intelligence that cannot be coerced into giving up its secrets and mysteries just because we want them.

That's why humbly approaching the body as a sacred and devoted act that you make to yourself is the only viable way to go. This sets the stage for your connection to your body and serves as the antidote to the transactional approaches we have grown accustomed to where we think this is about getting something. As in, *I do this and I get my body to do that*. This low-level way of relating to our bodies will only get us so far. Most of all, it will keep us from knowing that this is not about getting anything. Nor is it about tricking our bodies into anything.

Instead, it is about 'being with.' But in a time of instant access and the ten-easy-step culture, 'being with' feels too slow and effortful. It's not immediate enough. We want things. *Now*. Yet the pace of our bodies is slow and it takes time for things to reveal and to heal.

We have been conditioned to expect that everything comes to us immediately and easily. But our bodies and our connection to them are not something we order online that arrives the next day. Being with our bodies requires an ongoing, daily commitment. Progress, change or healing can be incremental and nearly invisible at times. Most of the body's vital processes happen below the surface, but that doesn't mean it's not working exactly as designed.

Remembering that there is a built-in connection to know what we truly need can give us the strength we require to commit to a lifelong, friendly and loving relationship with our own body.

CREATING THE SPACE

If you do one thing, *and one thing only*, to begin the journey of learning how to trust your body and make good choices, it would be this:

**Dedicate regular time and space to yourself
as a cornerstone of a lifelong apprenticeship to
learning how to trust your own body.**

As I began my own journey, I committed to a regular space and time for myself and it soon became second nature for me to notice when something felt 'off.' Even if I didn't know what it was, or what to do about it initially. It was like following breadcrumbs through the forest of my own body. Each crumb was significant in its ability to take me to the next place, until at some point, there I was! With myself, understanding something I had not before.

Creating space for myself has, *and always does*, leave me closer than ever to my body and to my ability to trust it. It sets the stage to see beyond all of the confusing and painful messages of the culture and a past that did not teach me the value of self-care, and into a caring and trusting relationship with myself instead.

Believe it or not, once you make the commitment to create space for yourself, it's not that hard. It doesn't require hours and hours. Though likely, the more time you spend with yourself, the more you'll want to do it. You don't need a membership or fancy equipment or even a special appointment. *Instead, it's just you, making you, and the space you need, a priority.*

It does not matter how, when or where you do it. Just that you do it. Maybe it's a formal practice like yoga or meditation. Maybe it's writing in a journal. Perhaps it's rising before everyone else and sitting at your kitchen table with a cup of tea and your own thoughts. It can be as simple as going for a walk or stepping outside to breathe the night air. It could be turning the radio off when you're driving to give yourself a chance to be with your own thoughts and feelings. Whatever it may be, *do something and do it regularly*. Consistency is key.

For many of us, this can require one of those enormous flat earth-round earth shifts that takes us from believing that taking time for ourselves in this way is selfish, to the reality that it is exactly the opposite of that. *Being in a body that is well cared for is the most generous act you will ever do for not only yourself, but for everyone around you.* So, when you notice all the excuses that come up around not being able to make the time for yourself, see them for what they are. *Excuses.*

BEFRIENDING

Simply put, befriending is the act of becoming a friend to yourself. This is one of the most powerful attitudes you can cultivate on The Embodied Journey, and it requires a decision on your part to stick with yourself, and to be good to yourself, through good times and bad.

This one shift alone changes everything. No matter what does or does not happen in your body. No matter what is there, or not. For as soon as you turn towards the body in a friendly way, *something immediately changes.*

Tears of relief may arise. A necessary surrender or insight may appear. Years of tension may begin to dissolve. Criticism's edge may lift. Closeness with another may result. Befriending will in all likelihood require an unraveling from all of the ways you have been unsupportive to yourself. You may even encounter a fair amount of grief as you experience just how hard and unfair you've been to yourself. Just know that this is to be expected, and is a natural part of the process. So count on it, and continue to be a friend to yourself as you discover all the ways you have not been a good friend.

An attitude of befriending yourself as a lifelong practice is to embark on a journey to a new shore, and then to rest in a place you have actually known all along. A place where you can trust what you know. A place that is kind. A place that is now available to you because you are not beating yourself up. *A place where the uncertainty and travails of life in a body are not only welcome, but are held with great reverence and respect.*

At its very best,

being in your body is an

agreement you make with

yourself to fully, and with

great reverence,

inhabit yourself.

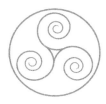

You Must Be in Your Body

"This body is made of earth and gold,
Sky and star, rivers and oceans,
Masquerading as muscle and bone."

- Radiance Sutras

To be in a body is to experience Life. *All of it*. It is to know ourselves. Our wholeness and our brokenness. Our divinity and our humanity. It is a doorway not only into experiencing the world, but also to what lies beyond. To be in a body is to love and be loved. To hurt and to be confused. It is to experience radiant moments of beauty, truth and connection, as well as ugliness, deceit and separation. At its very best, it is to be sovereign unto ourselves, while surrendering to Something More.

Your body is your first and most essential home. If you're not at home in your own body, not only will you not know what you need or how to care for yourself, you will never be at home in the world. Disconnected in this way, you will not know how to trust yourself; making you susceptible to the wrong choices and to beliefs and agendas that have nothing to do with what you truly need.

To be in a body is to walk a unique path that only you can walk. It is to find the courage you need for living all of its experiences, while claiming personal responsibility for how you meet up with life. *At its very best, being in your body is an agreement you make with yourself to fully, and with great reverence, inhabit yourself.*

A Harmful Separation

Fully inhabiting our bodies can be an enormous task in a world where there are so many distractions taking us away from ourselves. But every frightening issue we face these days has its origins in the individual and collective disconnection from the body of Truth that exists within the lived experiences of our bodies. When we are not in our bodies, we become separate from natural and life-promoting ways of living. What we think, say, do and choose becomes disembodied, and therefore destructive. Separate from the very ground that would tell us whether or not we are on track, we no longer know if what we are doing is helping or harming. We can no longer tell if we are honoring ourselves, *or not.*

All the ways that we're hurting as a species can be traced back to leaving our own bodies. Disconnected from ourselves, we create dis-ease and conflict with ourselves and others as we separate from what our lives truly need to be harmonious. And because we will always do to others what we do to ourselves, when we disengage from our bodies, we disengage from others. Including the very body that sustains us; the Earth herself.

In this state of separation from ourselves and others, we have no idea what we're doing to ourselves and others *because no one is home to experience it*. Not only that, perhaps the greatest damage of all is the individual and collective loss of joy, ease, pleasure, contentment and satisfaction of life in a body.

Unfortunately, disconnecting from our bodies, and from the bodies around us, is a 'normal' survival response to the overwhelm and trauma we all experience in a world that denies, commodifies, misuses and abuses the body. Dis-inhabiting ourselves in this way can initially be a sane response to insane, body-denying environments and painful histories.

But to live for a prolonged time outside of our very own skin leaves us vulnerable to the wrong things. We become destined to repeat over and over again habits and choices that do not work or feel good because we do not notice or feel we have any say over what is happening. Meaning, that the information the body is sending us to help us course correct, goes unnoticed and unheeded.

To be in a body is to live fully alive. To be disconnected from that same body is to inhabit the land of the walking dead. I know this might be hard to believe, but this is the good news. If the remedy for every troublesome thing you see around you is contained within you and your capacity to be at home in your own body with care, it means you have a choice. It means we all have a choice.

How we come to the experience of being in a body has the potential to change the world; changing not just your life but all the lives of those around you.

Therefore, learning to be more embodied is the very foundation of your health and well-being. It is the basis of your capacity to authentically and accurately assess what your genuine needs are while navigating the world. Embodiment is the road to gaining the self-trust you need that comes from being in a body and learning how to meet its needs. Knowing that when you are fully in your body, you can accurately perceive what it is asking for, along with what it does not want or need.

Seated in The Self

**To honor and satisfy real human needs is
to trust what your body is telling you.**

To trust your body is to trust yourself. To trust yourself
is to make life-giving choices for all. But in order to
learn how to do this, you must first be at home in your
own body. You must be present within yourself without
being distracted by the evaluations, criticisms and
busyness of daily life. You must value your whole self
without looking to others to tell you what to do. And
you must embrace your body beyond the perfectionism
and the preening of carefully curated selfies, and other
presentational depictions of yourself.

Ayurveda, the 5000-year-old healing tradition from
India, provides a definition of health that begins with
the premise of being *"seated in the Self."* Every time I
think of this, I get a visceral feeling of being centered,
grounded and located within my physical body, *and in
the deepest core of myself.* It feels like all of me is being recognized and included.

When I can sit in this place with myself, I am whole. No
longer fragmented or missing in my own life, I cease to
bring harm to myself or others. From this deeply
embodied wholeness, I can be with myself and contribute to the world in more loving, truthful ways than
when I am not at home in myself. For I can only be in

balance with all the bodies around me to the extent that I can be in balance with my own body.

Think of your body like a barometer that reads inner and outer conditions. With this crucial and timely information, you can better assess how to be here in the world because you have much more precise information about what you're experiencing; what you truly want, what to choose, what to believe in, what to move towards and what to move away from. This includes people, media, situations, substances, foods, work schedules and the types of medicine you use. Without this inner navigational system intact and appropriately honored, you are left stumbling your way through the confusing, overwhelming, distorted and intentionally seductive cultural messages that have nothing *whatsoever* to do with the real needs of life in your body.

Sadly, much of the advertising industry, along with our workplaces, bank on us not being at home in our bodies. This sets the stage for companies to sell us all kinds of things that we don't actually need. The same goes with the institutions we are a part of who can get more out of us productivity-wise when we are not home in our bodies. Not being attuned to our need for rest, regular mealtimes, fluctuating health states, bathroom trips or a sane human pace of living makes for very productive workers. But it's terrible when it comes to taking care of yourself.

LOCATING YOURSELF

Where am I right now? Am I here?

I find these two questions to be among the most important I can ask of myself throughout the day. It might sound ridiculously simple. Of course I'm here. *But am I?*

Too often, our bodies are in one place with our minds in another. This means we cannot be in relationship to what we're experiencing because *we're not there to experience it.* Split in this way, we live divided with the mind off in its fantasy land of past hurts, future worries and obsessions, while leaving the body without a present and clear mind to partner with. This leaves us in a perennial state of distraction; torn between what's real and what's not.

If you are not in your body at any given moment, how can you possibly know if what you're doing is working for you? Whether what you're doing is helping or harming? Whether what you are experiencing is even real or just a made-up fantasy of the mind?

> Bringing yourself back into the body is the work of a lifetime, and it is as simple as posing the questions: *Where am I right now? Am I here?*

Precious Gift or Commodity?

I teach yoga from the Kripalu tradition. The core teachings hold that the body is central and seminal to who we are. It's what we come back to moment by moment, both on and off the mat. The body is seen as an entry point to our connection to Divine Presence, as well as serving as the starting place for a healthy and happy life. Learning how to be in a body and take good care of it is seen as a precious gift you give to yourself, others and the world.

But this is not a perspective many of us hold when it comes to our bodies. Instead, we look at ourselves and wonder how we measure up to our culture's worship of youth, wealth and unattainable bodily 'ideals.' Many of us measuring our worth based on how many 'likes' we get on social media, while using filters to make us look better, thinner, younger, prettier.

Unfortunately, the sacred inhabitation of ourselves has been co-opted by selfies. Glam shots. Our push-up bra size. Our six-pack abs. Or whether or not we feel like the reflection in the mirror measures up to societal ideas about beauty, and therefore, value. These beliefs and others like them are nothing more than a destructive superficiality. Nothing more than an empty and rampant modern-day narcissism masquerading as satisfying embodiment.

To know what it is to be in your body takes time, strength and commitment, and is a deeply fulfilling experience that can only come from the inside-out, and that has nothing to do with what you can buy or what others expect of you. It calls for your compassion, tenderness and a quality of forgiveness for all the times you feel your body has let you down, or not measured up to some external standard. *Most importantly of all, being at home in your body demands owning up to what it actually is, while breaking away from what it is not.*

This requires navigating your way back into a body you have left, been chased out of or that has been co-opted by corporate America. It takes great skill to discern what your body actually is because we have come to see the body as the enemy; a foreign, awkward, uncomfortable, subpar, unruly and even scary place to inhabit. Perhaps we don't actually know what our bodies are because we're so busy trying to measure up to unrealistic beauty ideals. Or maybe you believe it isn't safe to be in a body or trust what you find there, and that's why you don't want to know it.

Departing can feel preferable and more secure for those of us not aware of the true nature of our bodies. Unfortunately, mainstream Western culture thrives on us being disconnected from ourselves in this way. Keeping us confused and doubtful about our bodies is a brilliant strategy for selling us things and getting more out of us productivity-wise. Look around at all that is available to keep you from being at home in your own body. Pot shops, liquor stores, streaming services, gambling, caffeine, junk food and more separate us from our bodies on a daily basis, and have become so common as to appear 'normal.'

The Antidote

Being in your body moment to moment, while learning the value of anchoring yourself there, is the antidote to all the disconnect. Choosing embodiment instead of the habitual ways we leave ourselves is key. Interestingly enough, staying with ourselves is exactly the opposite of what some of us think we should do. *Which is to leave*. So while it can be hard, sometimes *really* hard, to be with what you are experiencing, every single time you choose to do it, you are healing your relationship with yourself, and you're cultivating an experience of cherishing what your body really is. This will help you to become the one who embraces wherever you are on the journey, *no matter what.*

Which is why we're spending time here learning how to be more fully in a body, moment by moment and day by day. Every moment in life, even a small one, is a potent opportunity to discover what you really need, along with what it is that prevents you from giving yourself what you really need. What I'm talking about here is connecting more to *direct experience.* A way of being present so that you can fully tune into your body. This orientation serves as a corrective to the mis-attuned habits and beliefs we have developed. It also provides a trustworthy litmus test at any given moment.

I first came into contact with the practice of direct experience as a depth practitioner of yoga. I didn't come to yoga as a way to look better or even to manage stress. I got into it as a liberation practice to know the Truth of who I am and why I am here. What this has meant is coming into direct contact with a lot of mis-conceptions about my body. The 'direct experience' practice of being with everything that is happening in me continues to teach me about the conditioning and the belief systems I've taken on that have nothing to do with the truths of this body of mine.

Given how I grew up and the times we live in, this has included being with painful and sorrow-filled experiences. Yet this is precisely what I have needed most to heal the rupture in my relationship with my body. A kind of coming to terms with what is not true that has opened me up to levels of connection, intuition, self-trust, inner esteem and reverence for my life beyond anything I could have ever imagined.

During very intense retreats, practices and times in my life, I have returned to a question my teacher would pose, *"What is real and true in this moment?"* This simple question cuts through layers and layers of confusion, trauma, disconnection and mis-identification, helping me peel away false perceptions I have about myself, my body, and what I need most.

We all have untrue narratives about who we believe we are, what we need and what we most deserve. But when we turn to the question of what is real and true in any moment, instead of looking at ourselves through the lens of the past, we come into the reality of now. Meaning, we get to decide to continue on, or make a change. This is what I mean by direct experience. A way of knowing ourselves based on what is coming from the body *right now*, as opposed to the conditioning, fears and insecurities that train us to leave our bodily experience in an attempt to avoid being hurt again.

To put it another way, direct experience is about being present as a way to be fully in your body. We can call it direct experience, embodiment or mindfulness. By whatever name you use, this is about you being here. In your body. Now. *As is.* Whatever that means in any given moment. This is about you locating yourself in your body, and then honing your attention to stay anchored where you are. This can look like noticing your feet to the floor, your temperature, the way your clothes feel. Anything that reminds you of being in a body.

The Loving Observer

At its heart, this is *always* about learning to take the position of observing yourself as the loving observer of your own experience, or as some call it, the witness. This as opposed to the body shaming and condemnation of our inner judge and jury. But it takes determination to know yourself at this level. Being in a body, with all of its raw, unadulterated needs, can feel overwhelming, taking us right back to other times when we felt vulnerable in our bodies. This is why we *always* go at our own pace, and why *only we can determine that pace.* It is why we only go as fast as the slowest parts of us can go, allowing us to integrate each step forward, and why we have practitioners, practices and close confidantes we engage with for clarity and support.

Being in relationship with a body that houses tender and vulnerable places is a sacred responsibility. There are places within us that we do not want to bring more harm to. And yet, because of our human clumsiness and blindspots, we will inadvertently make some mistakes along the way. Take heart, the body does not expect perfection. It merely asks for our love, willingness and attention. Which is why forgiveness for ourselves, for what we can and cannot do, for what we have and have not done, is *mandatory*.

Forgiveness is the balm for any ridicule, censorship, shame or condemnation that comes up in you. For any harsh criticism that may come from others, and even, yourself.

A big revelation for me has been that yes, there are people from the past that I need to forgive, but it's most surprising how often it is *me* I need to forgive. For not knowing. For not doing better. For not living up to my own or other people's standards. For not...fill in the blank.

I often use an affirmation I got from the work of Louise Hay, that I modified to counteract my tendency to be too hard on myself. It goes like this:

I forgive you (my body) for not being what I wanted you to be.

I forgive you and I set you free.

I forgive you and I let you be.

This is a great one to use at the end of the day before bed or whenever you catch yourself getting down on yourself for not doing 'better.' Use it whenever something hurts or feels out of balance in your body that you feel like you had a hand in creating.

Conditioned as we have been to protect ourselves from past hurts, it can feel like danger is imminent when we touch back into the body and become present to what it needs. Which is why learning to pay greater attention to ourselves only works when we couple it with lots and lots of kindness, compassion and when needed, even self-protection. To do otherwise is to overexpose ourselves or turn an unfair and harsh light on ourselves without the balancing effects of understanding. That understanding being, we are all where we are for very good, and very sane reasons. *But perhaps now, you are ready to do something different?*

LETTING THE MUD SETTLE

I want to share with you a simple but profound way to be in your body, *as is*. Every morning, I begin my daily practice in the same way. I sit. I literally just sit. I breathe. I look out the window. I might sip hot water. But basically, I sit and do nothing.

What would possess a woman to do nothing?

The discovery that when all the mud settles, the mud being the difficult and troubling thoughts, emotions and bodily sensations threatening to take over, a sense of spaciousness washes over me; creating enough space for me to see, more clearly and effortlessly, *what is real and what is true.*

From this spaciousness, a greater connection to my body and its truths becomes available to me. This means that any problem I have, any solution I am seeking or any balm needed for my broken heart or suffering body, is there. *Always.*

I first discovered this practice when my mind would kick into high gear in an absolute frenzy over everything I needed and wanted to get done after my kids had gone off to school. My mind hounded me about how much I had to do and in what order, how fast and how well. It was maddening. So much so that I couldn't settle into yoga or meditation because the demands of my mind were that intense.

Initially I sat, doing nothing, in protest. It was my way of saying to the thoughts, *I want out. I am not playing anymore. I will not negotiate with you.*

And then, at some point, what began as an exasperated refusal to participate with an agitated mind, turned into a portal transporting me to a whole new universe I didn't even know was accessible with so little effort. It turns out, I didn't need to hack my way into the ease and peace I was seeking. It was already there.

Letting the mud settle does take time and some getting used to. Some days, it only takes a few minutes for everything to settle down. Other days, it takes a lot longer. Even on the days my mind pushes me to get going, to do something for god's sake, I know better now. I know that in doing nothing, everything I have ever hoped for will show up when given the space it needs.

So sit back. Keep your feet on the Earth. Feel the warmth of the sun or the coolness of the air. Let your breath be where you put your attention. Breathe in a way that allows your body to be big enough to include all of what you are experiencing in this moment.

Think of a candle melting and allow yourself to flow down in the same way. Follow that image over and over and over again until you feel weighted in a pleasant and settled way. When you feel like the mud has settled, even a little bit, notice what reveals itself to you by way of what is real and true in your body in this moment.

A little caveat. To the busy, stressed out, divided and fear-based mind this practice can feel like a death. It is. But it's only the death of things that need to go anyway. The death of anything you would be better off without; like all the ways that your mind is unfair and unkind to your body

as you unnecessarily fret over imagined problems. So when the mind screams and screams
and starts rolling out all the heavy artillery
around what a slacker-loser you are for not
doing more, nod your head and continue to sit,
knowing that when all the mud settles out, you
will be left at home in your own body.

Nothing is separate
from anything else
when it comes to
life in a body.

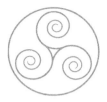

Body Basics

"Dealing with the truths of the body leads us to dealing with the truths of our lives and who we really are."

- Yoganand

Every day you decide how you want to feel based on how fully you breathe, what you eat, how well you sleep, who you're in relationship with and more. The good news is, the instructions for how to do all of this are encoded right into you. Use what follows as a reminder of what your body already naturally knows how to do when given the chance.

When my children were young, but old enough to venture out into the world beyond my reach, I knew I had to teach them something they could carry with them wherever they went. Something that would help them return to the wisdom of their bodies. Something that would help them stand in the face of too many life-depleting choices. So when they were old enough to know dessert was being offered at a party and asked me for it, I would say to them, *"What does your body say?"*

This is the opposite of what many of us often do. *Dessert? Of course!* Or perhaps...*Dessert? Never!* We reach for it without checking in to see how full we are, not noticing if we even like the taste of what's in our mouth. Disconnected from our body, we power through the last bite, even after we've had enough. Or maybe, dessert would be a great choice in the moment, but we never, *ever,* allow it to be an option because that would mean we were being overly indulgent, weak or 'bad.'

How often have you already decided what you'll choose to do in regard to your body before the moment ever arrives? How many automatic reactions do you engage in without checking in with your body first? Without wondering, *What does my body say?* Without checking in with our bodies first, we leave the habit-driven, conditioned mind and the social pressures around us, in charge. The voices that insist, *dessert is desirable* or *dessert is not allowed,* without allowing our bodies and what they need to be the deciding factor.

The trouble is, when we do not check in with our bodies first, we impose upon them what they do not need or want. Maybe even, *what might bring harm.*

Have you ever wondered how your life would change if you checked in with your body first? If you asked its opinion around the choices you were making. *Might you eat differently? Go to bed when you're tired? Slow down? Rest more? Recognize that the endless scrolling is actually leaving you dissatisfied and miserable? Learn to set a healthy boundary around who you're spending time with? See that the way you're medicating yourself each night actually doesn't feel that good to you?*

Bodies that don't get what they *really* need, never feel good.

Not feeling good in your body will have consequences far beyond tiredness, pain and illness. Living in a body whose most basic needs are not recognized and honored is to live deprived in body, mind, soul and relationship. It is to lack the vitality and the commitment necessary to be in the world in a vital and healthy way. It is to live hungry; starved of what you really need. Worst of all, *it is to live as if you don't deserve better.*

The good news is, you don't have to go out and get anything. Feeling good in your body doesn't require special clothes or an expensive program. You only need a willingness to turn towards an inner wisdom that wants nothing more than to express itself in healthy ways. Best of all, this state of being is as close to you as becoming aware of your most basic biological urges like hunger, thirst, elimination and sleep. It's not glamorous or flashy and it might not get a lot of 'likes,' but by tuning into the basics of your most essential needs, you will not only feel better, you will empower yourself in your ability to know what you need; giving you the most exquisite navigational system *ever* to move through a world with too many seductive and health-depleting options.

Set an intention each day to be at home in your body as often as you can, while learning to listen to the 'mundane' daily needs of your embodiment. With this kind of attention, you're back in connection with a deep and abiding Intelligence that wants only to support you. This is something that belongs to you and that is far more than another health program, or someone else's opinion. This is built into you, and is as near to you as recognizing and honoring your next bodily need, like going to the bathroom when you need to, drinking when you're thirsty, putting the fork down when you're full.

Because you have so many needs throughout each and every day, you literally have dozens and dozens of opportunities to practice. Don't be fooled by the simplicity of this. *Satisfying real human needs is an inside job*, and is the exact opposite of where many of us go to figure out what the body is asking for. While it may take time for you to adjust to a new way of being in your own skin, know this: *Each time you can land in your body, listening to what it is telling you, you are one step closer to claiming sacred responsibility for your health and well-being.*

This *way of being* with the body's most basic needs has nothing to do with having the right gear, following a celebrity diet, downloading the newest app or trying the latest exercise fad. Instead, it is a way of inhabiting yourself that puts you and your body at the very center of each and every choice you make.

While not always easy, holding this awareness is not complicated. It's as basic as this: *Do you know when something doesn't feel good, or is not working for your body?* If you can connect to this feeling, you are on your way. Tuning in to what does not feel good is a barebones way to begin. While it might sound paradoxical, if you can allow yourself to feel what doesn't feel good, you are at an authentic starting point. And if you can be willing to stay with that without judgment, if you can be willing to dig a little deeper, something will reveal itself to you, about you and what it is that keeps you from giving your body what it wants and needs.

Getting Even More Real With Yourself

How often do you do something to your body that does not feel good to you? Maybe it's eating and drinking too much or ingesting the wrong things for your constitution. Maybe it's not getting enough sleep or satisfying movement each and every day. Perhaps it's using sugar or caffeine to perk the body up, only to go through the inevitable crash later in the day.

Why do you think you do this?

This is not about judgment or insinuation. It's an honest question asked to help you get real with yourself as you uncover what's beneath some of the choices you make. Forget about finding a quick fix or ready-made answers and instead, be with the question. Be with the feelings that arise in you. This is what turned things around for me back in my twenties. The willingness to notice how what I was doing was hurting me, and then the courage to look a little deeper.

Spend time noticing yourself, especially when what you're doing is not working for you. Be curious. Be understanding. Suspend judgment. If you can pay attention to what is not working, while staying open in the spirit of discovery, self-love and devotion to your own life, something very important will reveal itself to you.

In the end, the finest litmus test will always be your ability to be in your body, responding to what it needs. Your direct experience of what is happening in your body transcends expert advice, fads, what influencers are peddling and any other agendas that are not in alignment with the truest needs of a human being. Don't try to change your lifestyle choices all at once. Pick one area in your life that's not working, and begin there.

Eventually, whatever unmet need you focus on will lead you to all the rest because *everything is connected*, and what you do in one part of your life, you do for all of your life. Each time you choose to be in your body, listening to what it needs, each time you act on that knowing, you teach yourself how to respond to yourself in authentic and integrity-filled ways.

How Needs Get Distorted Early On

Human needs, and our ideas about what they are and how to satisfy them, date all the way back to infancy and childhood. In the beginning, we were purely need-based beings. A need was met by our caretakers. *Or it wasn't.* Without any self-consciousness, we expressed our needs for the whole world to hear and see. Sometimes we received the response we most needed. And sometimes, *we didn't.*

In the beginning, we had no sense of feeling bad about having needs. We knew nothing about subverting, hiding or diminishing what our bodies most yearned for. Being brand new to the world and these bodies of ours, we counted on those around us to decipher and meet our basic and non-negotiable biological demands. We did this without a thought or worrying about how it would be received.

Having needs and expressing them was completely natural. We learned early on to make sense of the world based on what was happening in our bodies, and the responses we got. That's why it can feel so murky or charged now when it comes to how we do, *or do not*, meet our most basic daily needs. It's all tied up in childhood, and what we did or did not get. Based on what happened growing up sets the template for beliefs around whether we deserve to have our needs met. *If our needs are even allowed to exist.*

To be clear, I am not just talking about the 'big' moments only of abuse or neglect. Our needs getting distorted shows up in the most mundane moments of life like when someone told you to put a coat on when you weren't cold. Or when you were forced to eat what was on your plate. Or when you were told to smile and be nice to someone who did not feel good for you to be around.

No matter what the experience, this is a very, *very* tender place to be with; born from a time well before we had the words to understand why we may have gotten, or not gotten, what we did or did not want or need. But without including this potentially difficult piece of life, it will matter not what new diet or 'full-proof' exercise program you try if you don't understand that the root cause of why you struggle to take good care of yourself is linked to deep internal beliefs around whether or not you feel like you even deserve to be cared for.

We all have our stories and beliefs about our needs not being met and all the unfulfilling substitutions we accept in their stead. Maybe we learned to be someone who did not have needs because that made us appear strong, reliable and independent. Maybe we subjugate our needs for others, believing this is how we get love or that by putting others first gives us an escape hatch from having to deal with our own unmet requirements. Or maybe we act overly needy as a way to keep others close.

We have so many reasons for never making a wave, issuing a demand or having any kind of need that might even slightly inconvenience another, or, god forbid, rock the boat of the status quo. How often have you accepted, with a smile even, what you did not need or want? How often have you been locked in fear around speaking a real need to another? Or how about being patently unaware that you actually have a choice around how your needs are expressed and met?

You might even be thinking, *Needs? What needs? What are you talking about? I'm fine!* Fear. Shame. Indulgence. Guilt. Resistance. Secrecy. Round and round it goes in the deep places of our unconscious mind around satisfying basic human needs. But here's the real deal. As children, we were purely biologically-driven, need-based beings. We had no story. No unworthiness, distortion or manipulation. All we experienced was whether a need was present *or not*. Whether a need was satisfied. *Or not*.

I am in no way minimizing or discounting how painful it can be to not have been met as children. What I am saying is that no matter what happened, know this: *Your body was born with natural needs built right into you. These needs serve as the center of a powerful guidance system that lets you know how to care for yourself, and how to be in the world. They are not negotiable, they are not someone else's to take care of at this point in your life and they are not amenable to what someone is trying to get you to do or ignore.*

Your needs are not for sale and are not to be overlooked for someone else's comfort.

As adults our job now is to find a way to return to the innate Intelligence we were born with. We do this by learning to be at home in our bodies, by occupying ourselves so fully that we make room for all the needs that may have gotten squashed, distorted and waylaid. We do it by giving ourselves all the time, permission and patience we need to make our way back home to ourselves. We do it by seeing that everything, *and I do mean everything*, is an opportunity to get closer and closer to honoring yourself and what you most need. Mistakes, uncertainties and frustrations included.

TUNING IN

To affirm to yourself that you do know what you need, that it is in fact built into you, try this simple gesture to your body each morning to remind yourself of what you already know, but may have forgotten. *Or never learned to begin with.*

Before getting out of bed in the morning, pause for as long as you can to feel for what's happening in your body. Before the busy, rational mind kicks into overdrive with all the things you must get to, stay where you are just breathing and be with your body. When you feel settled enough, and the moment feels right, ask your body:

How are you doing?

What do you need?

Don't move until you hear, sense or feel an answer.

Don't be fooled by the simplicity of this moment. *It is powerful beyond words to be in a body and know how to figure out what it needs.* More than anything else, this takes your time and your devotion to tune in to yourself as you listen way down deep for what's there, and for what's being asked.

When you do this, imagine yourself in two parts. There is the baby body of you just needing what it needs, and there is the grown-up body of you who can now meet those needs. But in order for you to attune to what this baby body of yours is needing, without the overlay of judgment, shame or impatience, you must be willing to come to yourself without having all the answers, without having to fix anything and without needing to shut anything up.

Needs Exist for Good Reason

To disregard the signals of your body's most basic biological requirements is to create dis-ease and hardship in every area of your life. Real biological needs exist within you for a reason. They owe their allegiance to no one but you and have no agenda other than to be met. Simply put, the basic needs of the body are a set of non-negotiable prerequisites for health, without the satisfaction of which your body, and therefore your life, *will not work.*

With this understanding in mind, we're ready to dive into some guidelines around what a body actually needs to thrive. What comes next is meant to serve as a kind of template to help get you started. This is by no means a full treatment on the topic. That would fill volumes. I am being intentionally sparse here to give you plenty of room to explore on your own because providing you with too much information will hinder the experience of you getting to know yourself from the inside-out.

Enjoy, and let this be part of your lifelong apprenticeship on becoming the expert of your body's most basic needs.

Here they are:
- *The Breath*
- *Hydration*

- *Real Food*
- *Rest*
- *Movement*
- *Good Company*
- *Connection*

Simple, huh? If it sounds too basic, that's the point. We've got it all wrong when we complicate what the body's real needs are. But don't take my word for it. Explore this for yourself. You might even hold the question, *What if it's really true that my health and well-being is as basic and straightforward as this?*

This doesn't mean we don't have bad habits, mental conditioning, problematic beliefs, cultural pressures and more to unpack. We do. It just means that to get clear about what we seem to be so confused about, we must start in the right place. Otherwise, our efforts will be to no avail, we will be subject to false promises and we will be left feeling bad, *yet again*, because we know we should take better care of ourselves, but somehow just can't get there.

Try this. When you get up in the morning and you're getting ready for your day, ponder how it is that you want to feel today. *Which choices will bring you closer to that experience?* And which ones further away? While there are choices that are most certainly more supportive or less than others, this is never about being right or wrong, good or bad. Instead, it is about being with yourself in an honest and compassionate way as you figure out, through trial and error, what works for you.

Practically speaking, it breaks down like this:

- *Do you know when you're hungry or thirsty and can you nourish yourself accordingly?*

- *Do you know when you're tired and can you allow yourself to rest?*

- *Do you know when it feels good or not to be in the company of another and can you give yourself permission to act on that?*

- *Do you know how to move your body in a way that feels good to you?*

- *Does your body breathe freely and deeply?*

- *Do you feel like you're part of Something Bigger that gives your life meaning and purpose?*

- *Do you get outside every day and take it all in?*

Use these questions to get curious about yourself and what you really and truly need. These are not admonitions to make yourself feel even more shame and guilt. They are provocative questions that can help you remember the basics of who you are and what it takes to nourish your body. Let them work on you over time. As in, a lifetime. Let the questions move you beyond right and wrong and instead, let them take you back home to your body.

Pick a question to work on for a while. Use the question as a prompt, a wondering, a source of inspiration, but never as a way to beat yourself up with. Be on the look-out for what gets in the way of you living these questions. Include the obstacles, for they provide life-giving guidance that we can miss out on if we deny or judge what gets in the way.

A Powerful Question

All of this reminds me of a question a teacher once posed. She asked, *"Could we consider participating with the truest rhythms and needs of our bodies?"* What a stunning question! And what a great way to sum up what we're talking about here. Instead of thinking in terms of diets, being 'good,' exercising and the like, could you get into the habit of participating with your body in such a way that you aligned with its real needs?

To give you an example of *what this is not*, consider a commercial I once saw where the tagline read: *The future of health is on your wrist*. The screen showed a frenzied woman operating at warp speed as dictated to her by the device she was wearing on her arm. It commanded,

Relax. Then, *Run, Swim, Do Tae Kwon Do, Dance*. I watched in horror as she manically leapt from one instruction to the next like a puppet hopped up on adrenaline. All directed by a tiny machine strapped to her arm.

There was absolutely no participating here with the true rhythms and needs of her body. If this weren't so alarming, it would be funny. *Saturday Night Live* parody funny.

But it's not funny. Not when you consider how many of us are learning to take our bodily cues and the fulfillment of its needs and expressions, from electronic devices. Not funny at all when you see how many of us are perfectly comfortable taking health advice from people and corporations trying to sell us something. The same ones, by the way, trying to keep us insecure and doubtful about our ability to be in our bodies without them, as they make money off those same insecurities and fears.

The image I've just described suggests that we must listen to instructions from a piece of machinery to know what we need. The underlying premise being that our ability to read our own body is so beyond us that it's best to outsource our wisdom to something non-human. Something more infallible. This is a sad example of us being caught up in the wrong things because we're not in our bodies, and because we don't actually know what they need.

Do you know what I think? I think the real future of health is YOU. Your built-in capacity to care for yourself, fully restored and acted upon. Your inner and personal guidance trusted above all else. Because here's the truth, when the basics of your body are met, *everything works better.* Your health. Your relationships. Your self-esteem. Your mood. Your happiness.

If you're familiar with Maslow's Hierarchy of Needs, you know what I mean. Until human needs like food, shelter and safety are met, we cannot ascend to the joys, beauty, self-acceptance and self-knowledge that all of us not only yearn for, but that is our birthright and that is readily available to us when we take the time to tend to the body's most basic needs.

The Common Sense of the Body

At the beginning of every college semester with my classes, I would tell students that what we would be doing together would be simple, common-sense approaches. Obvious things about the body that we often don't pay attention to, or know to pay attention to. So obvious, that it's easy to miss or discount.

Based on their initial responses (as well as feedback at the end of the course) I often got the sense that some of them believed me to be the village idiot. Some naive fool or New Age hippie believing that we can influence what is happening in our bodies in some hocusy-pocusy way.

But after more than fifteen years of working with students in this way, I am more convinced than ever that what it takes for us to live our lives well is indeed quite simple, and extraordinarily obvious. Not necessarily easy, but absolutely available to each and every one of us. But because our culture has become so accustomed to making things more complicated than it needs to be, along with our proclivity to believe that the fix exists outside of ourselves, what I'm proposing here can feel to some anywhere from naive to downright dangerous. *But it is neither.*

Over the years, the number of students who shifted or resolved long standing mental, emotional and physical conditions was astounding! *How did they do it?* By tending to the basic needs of the body. When they did, changes occurred in anxiety, depression, headaches, muscle pain, insomnia, panic attacks, digestive disorders, allergies, self-esteem issues, relational challenges and more, 'just' by giving their bodies what they most needed.

What all of this has taught me is that until the basics of the body are met, not only will health and happiness elude us, we will not have an accurate picture of what is happening in the body if it gets sick. For until the essential basics of the body are satisfied, nothing works as it should. Not digestion, not immune functioning, not the muscles, heart or anything else for that matter.

Throwing pills and procedures at a body without stopping to consider what it really needs us to do, *or stop doing*, we mask the root causes of whatever is causing the imbalance. Without this as a starting point, we will not be addressing what actually needs addressing. Which means, *we will not heal*. No amount of aspirin will properly address headaches that arise from tension or from eating foods that your body is allergic to. No amount of cholesterol medication will make up for the Standard American Diet or a sedentary life. Nor will you find a sleeping pill that truly resolves the insomnia that arises from unchecked stress or a life devoid of meaning and purpose.

Taking this one step further, whatever form of health-care you do use is rendered less effective when the most basic needs of your body, the very building blocks of health and well-being itself, have not been met. *No external fix will ever make up for this*. You can take all the multivitamins you want, but if you don't feed yourself real food, your body will lack energy, have trouble eliminating, sleeping and concentrating. You can use all the health apps you want, but if you don't feel like who you are and what you do matters, you will not see the results being promised to you.

No Outside Rules Here

As far as I'm concerned, there is no one system that can tell all of us how to care for ourselves. Which is why you will find no rule here about how many hours you should sleep. No prescription that you should lift weights or walk three times a week. Nothing said about eating dairy or not. No external standard to be met. This may feel heretical to all the expert advice you get, or maybe like too much personal responsibility to take on. I say, so be it.

**Meeting real human needs is an inside job,
knowing how to do it is wired into you,
and it is only yours to do.**

Does it take time to become skilled at connecting to your body and what it needs? Yes. Are there things you will have to change and let go of? *Absolutely.* But do you, do any of us, really need a constant barrage of disembodied outside information? I would say no.

Get some basic facts, and I do mean basic, on how a body works from a source that is not trying to be the know-it-all in your health. Find people who can support you and who are practicing what they preach. If you catch a whiff of someone imposing their ideas on you without including your wise body in the equation, or if you find yourself looking for a quick fix or abdicating personal responsibility, you might want to rethink your choice.

It's only human to want immediate answers to what ails us. To want the fix RIGHT NOW. It can be so easy to judge ourselves for not knowing better. For finding it hard to admit that what we're doing isn't working. *That maybe it never really has.* But if you can set all of that aside, you are in the position of starting anew with your body and what it needs. From there, you can take that first step towards figuring out what it is you really need with your next step on the journey being as close to you as the next decision you make about what to give your body.

Do that over and over and over again. *Every single day.* Be willing to give your body the time it needs to soak in the experience of its needs being met, and from there, *so much is possible.*

THE 'ABSOLUTES'

What could I absolutely not live without when it comes to my body?

We live in a world filled with so many wants, and so many people trying to sell us what they believe we 'should' want. But to be in alignment with our truest selves, and therefore the world, is to intentionally tune into *the real needs* of your body. The ones that are timeless and universal. The ones that are there whether you are a man or a woman, whether you live in the northern hemisphere or the southern part of the planet. Whether you were born in this time period or another one entirely.

Consider this a not-so-little thought experiment where you allow your mind to range far and wide when it comes to what you really and truly need to not only survive, but to thrive in your body in the purest sense of that word. A good way to do this is to imagine what you must have needed as a baby that was non-negotiable. This helps to break through the confusion between real needs and any wants generated by the times we are living in or by distortions of the past.

The experience of being at home in your body and listening for what it needs will feel different day to day, will often not be what you expected, and at some point will feel far better to be doing, *than not*. At home in your real needs, you begin to access a kind of wisdom that transcends what other people think you should do, what marketers are selling to you, any fears that keep you small and what any other body-splitting agendas of the times are pushing. In the end, bringing you back home to yourself where at home in yourself, you are at home in the world.

So, what could you absolutely not live without when it comes to your body?

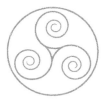

You Must Be Willing to Learn the Language of Your Body

"Symptoms are you, telling you, about you."

- Kelly Brogan

Your body is Intelligent and it knows how to heal. Symptoms and sensations are the language of the body offering you essential and valid information about your life. Bodily imbalances do not happen in isolation and they are not a punishment or evidence of wrongdoing.

I once heard a physician say that if you spent enough time with a patient, they would tell you *what's wrong, how they got there and what they need.* Wow! Can you imagine our mainstream medical system practicing medicine with that in mind? How incredibly accurate and visionary to place a person's perspective about themselves, along with the wisdom contained within them, at the very center of their care.

Can you imagine a world of health and healing where each of us knew what was wrong with our bodies, how we got there and what we needed? The ripple effects would extend well beyond the health of our bodies and into *every single facet* of what it means to be alive.

Believe it or not, it's possible for you to know yourself at this level, and for you to find practitioners who honor and respect that innate knowing and capacity in you. That's exactly what we're working towards here on The Embodied Journey. You, possessing that level of connection, awareness and confidence about what's happening in your own body, along with your ability to choose health practitioners, *whatever their discipline*, who recognize this in you as *the prerequisite* for creating health, healing and embodied thriving within you.

Yours to Do

This way of being in your body includes all of you, and is yours to protect and initiate in the work you do with yourself and others around your health. This is you and your body being at the center of the choices you make around health. This is radically different from being relegated to the periphery of your health care, where technologies, insurance codes or a one-size-fits-all medicine takes center stage instead of you and your needs.

This perspective recognizes that everything in your life is connected, important and therefore, *must be included*. This includes the recognition that imbalances in your body do not happen in isolation, or even overnight, but in the context of your whole life. This includes your thoughts, emotions, habits, relationships, work life, cultural heritage, past and more that are all playing a contributing role in your health and well-being.

As true and valid as this perspective is, it will never be handed to you by another, or by the systems currently in place. Instead, *it is something you must claim*. At its heart, this is about taking the steadfast position that you deserve better than to be told that what you think doesn't matter. That you deserve better than assembly line healthcare. That you deserve better than to be treated like a child. T*hat you are worth the time and effort it takes to get a full picture of who you are, what is happening for you and what it is that you most need.*

This means allowing yourself to begin exactly wherever it is that you find yourself with the symptoms, states and signals of your body while giving yourself the space, time and support that you need to move through your own unique experiences in your own way.

This will not always be easy to do. As a culture, we love to pathologize, catastrophize, outsource and vilify the body and what it's doing. We make our bodies wrong and tell ourselves that every problem we have will lead to dire consequences. Which only serves to terrify and infantalize us. Or we go in the other direction by ignoring and denying the body's genuine needs. Or we commodify it by believing that health is the same as looking young according to some unachievable image of technological perfection.

As we get older, it can get worse as we begin to embrace the 'wear and tear' narrative, expecting everything to break down. Which then of course requires a bucket of pills to manage this decrepit body of ours, while we bond with others over how many things hurt and what no longer works. Most of all, because we have come to believe that the language of the body is beyond our understanding, we always need someone else to translate its symptoms to tell us what is going on inside of our very own bodies.

Becoming Present Enough to Listen

Listening to what your body is communicating requires, first and foremost, *that you are in your body*. Otherwise, how will you know what's happening? How will you accurately decipher the messages being sent? The practices from the chapter *You Must Be in Your Body* (or anything else that you do to be more embodied) can help you begin to remedy the avoidance and the mistrust we can experience about life in a body we are not actually in. Never mind, *not listening to.*

Being in your body is the first step to developing a trusting relationship with the messages your body is sending you, and is something that requires lots of time, devotion and care. Without this, you're likely to get your signals crossed by trying to receive messages from a body you're not actually in. This will leave you confused and convinced that you can't interpret what the body is telling you. That's why I can't overstate how essential it is that you make the intention to inhabit your body on a regular basis.

Once you're in your body, the next step is to become aware of the words you use to speak to yourself and others about your body. Choosing your words mindfully when speaking about this precious body of yours and what it is doing, *is a must.* How we name anything matters. Using honest and compassionate descriptions is an essential starting point for more accurately understanding what your body is experiencing. Using pejorative, fear-based and negative phrases about your body obscures your ability to experience it clearly which renders any 'observations' you make about it, *inaccurate.* False statements and ideas will take you to unhelpful, maybe even harmful solutions because you have mis-named your symptoms and bodily experiences.

Without understanding the full significance of your body's messages, how could you possibly know what needs to be done to restore your health and wellbeing? *Most of all, ongoing negativity towards and about your body has a detrimental impact on your overall experience of being alive.* In other words, *it just won't feel good to be here.* Not to mention that cutting edge sciences in the fields of the mind-body connection have been demonstrating for decades that your thoughts do in fact impact your health. *One way or another.*

Becoming more conscious about the language you use when it comes to your body is about developing a more precise (not perfect) ability to name the moment to moment truth of life in your body. Your ability to cultivate this language will determine how well you can respond to what the body is saying, along with what it needs.

Creating an Embodied Love Language

When my mother was still alive, we had this bit we would do. She would disparage some part of her body. Usually, it was her stomach that was never flat enough because of the four cesareans and one hysterectomy. Other days it would be the skin that was too loose because she was in her eighties or her weight on any given day that she tracked by daily weigh-ins on the bathroom scale.

When she spoke to herself negatively, I would look at her and tilt my head. To which she would respond, *"Oh yeah, I'm not supposed to say that."*

It was funny. *And not.* After years of us doing this bit together, she knew that if she criticized her body in my presence, I was going to challenge her. I don't think she ever fully understood the extent of what she was doing to herself. I don't think she ever allowed herself to feel the impact of maligning her body, sometimes *with great disgust* at its inability to measure up to some externalized state of perfection. I don't think she ever got it was her own self she was disgusted by.

Your body is listening, and the words you use about it hurt or heal.

If this makes sense to you, practice being more mindful about the phrases you use in reference to your own body. When you catch yourself using hurtful words, say, *I'm sorry. I take that back.*

While science is finally catching up to the ways that our thoughts impact our physical health, I urge you not to wait. Start now. Be as kind to your own body as you would be to someone you dearly loved, and I will guarantee you something; a whole lot of the mental and emotional hurt and suffering will vanish. And there is a very good chance that something in your physical health will shift as well.

The Language of Your Body

Beyond the specific words we use to reference our bodies, there is a language of the body that is different from the thoughts, ideas and beliefs of the rational mind. It is a continuous stream of information in the form of urges, sensations and symptoms that is speaking to you *every moment of every day*. But if you are not aware that these bodily experiences are a language, you won't understand its messages, and you'll need others to tell you what to do with your own body.

This does not mean we don't seek assistance from wise counsel to help us figure out our body's messages. But it does mean that because we are the only ones inside this body of ours, we must be able to tune into what it is saying so that we are starting with the right information. Your ability to focus into bodily states and sensations helps you become more fluent in the language of your body, which then gives you access to invaluable information as to what to pay attention to and what to ignore. What's important and what doesn't matter at all. What is possible and what is not. What you have jurisdiction over, and what is out of your hands.

Think about it. How can you ask the right questions, accurately respond or seek the best approaches, if you don't know how to tune into your own experience? Without the right questions, how can you find the right answers? Without tuning into this world of bodily information, how do you know whether what you are doing is helping or hurting? Or if your 'solutions' are exacerbating the very problem you are trying to heal?

Or maybe even causing a whole new set of problems which then kicks off doubt, shame, frustration and disappointment as you circle round and round the wrong approaches. Approaches that may never bring the relief you seek because you did not start with an accurate assumption to begin with.

Every symptom, sensation, instinct and urge of your body is part of a necessary and adaptive mechanism that allows you to adjust, stop, do something, know something, survive and ultimately thrive. *Does it make any sense to you that you would have no ability to understand these messages, or that they were only an inconvenient and unruly voice to quell?*

From a purely survival perspective, does it make any sense that you would be unable to make good use of the communications you're receiving without an outside expert interpreter? How would we survive as a species without a built-in understanding of our very own bodies and what they're saying?

From a common sense, survival-based, mammalian-self-care-is-built-in perspective, there is no validity whatsoever to the belief that the body's communications are problematic, need to be silenced or are someone else's domain; despite the widespread acceptance of this narrative in the culture. I'll take this one step further. Holding false sets of assumptions about the body's signals and how they need to be approached undermines your health and well-being; eroding your ability to trust yourself, while degrading your capacity to claim personal responsibility. *This is as problematic to healthy embodiment as believing that the earth is flat was to our sense of the world and how it worked.*

This can feel like an enormous mental shift to make in such technologically-laden times, where the inventions of the human mind reigns supreme over the 'foreignness' and the unpredictability of the body, and where bodily signals can feel too complicated, messy or frightening to be with. Where doubt, uncertainty and fear have replaced a basic sense of trust and belonging in the body.

But think about it. Does it make any sense to you that we would be built to not understand or know how to respond to the communications of the body? Does it make sense to believe that symptoms are an annoyance to get away from or something to be terrified of, as opposed to valid information?

**Our bodies are wise and
what they are saying has meaning.**

But given our current love affair with technology-centered medicine, so absolute in its promotion of infallible scans, tests and information, trusting the body in this way may seem naive. *Dangerous even.* But if you consider that the bodies we inhabit biologically hale from a time before all these interventions, does it not make sense that Nature would have built right into us ways to hear, understand and respond to information coming from our very own bodies? That we might be well-served to refer to the millions of years of evolution that have gotten us here?

If you're new to learning the language of your body, it's really no different from learning a new language or brushing up on your native tongue when you haven't spoken it in a while. It takes time and practice. But as with anything else in life, the more you do it, the better you get. Until one day, you find that you're fluent. This doesn't happen overnight (which can be hard to hear in a world with a magic-bullet mentality), but each step you take brings you closer to a deep and abiding honoring and trusting of the body you call home.

Welcoming in What You Don't Want

During a somatic training I once did, the teacher introduced one of the simplest, yet impactful attitudes I have ever taken with myself. He suggested that when something arose in us (for our purposes here, something in the body) instead of pushing it away or being upset by it, simply saying instead, *"Welcome. It's okay that you're here."*

I know this sounds ridiculous. *Why would you ever welcome in what you did not want?* This approach is not saying you want 'bad' things in the body to stay, or that you even like what is happening. It's saying, *I recognize you're here. I am not denying or twisting away from your existence. I welcome you in the spirit of meeting up with reality and self-discovery.*

Meeting yourself in this way allows you to call what is going on by its real and true name, putting you in the position to hear what is being spoken to you. It is only from a place of welcoming in that you are ready to hear the language of your body, and all that it offers you by way of navigating the changing states of life in a body.

Aligning with the wisdom of sensations, urges, instincts and symptoms allows you to recognize what is happening within you, even when you don't want it. Even when you're not completely sure about what to do. Even when you can't articulate your experience or when others don't understand or agree with what you're doing. Instead, welcoming in what is there puts you in the position of knowing *what's wrong, how you got there and what you most need.*

While there is no guarantee I can give when it comes to learning the language of your body, no certainty I can offer, I can say this: *When you choose to be in your body and welcome in its communications, your relationship to your body, to health, to others and to the entire world will dramatically shift for the better.* And it all begins by fully showing up for what your body is saying, and by learning to believe that what your body is doing has meaning and is worthy of your time, attention and yes, *even your devotion.*

A DAILY PAUSE

Get in the habit of pausing at least once a day. Take a long, slow, breath and ask yourself, *What am I feeling right now in my body?* Name what you are sensing out loud, just like you would practice repeating phrases out loud in a language course.

Pay attention to the parts of the body involved and the quality of the sensations you're experiencing. Dull. Sharp. Surface. Penetrating. Fleeting. Long-Standing. This is not about letting the mind impose worries and fears on top of the experience the body is having. *Instead, can you just be with what is happening by simply naming what is there, while you put aside the negative interpretations of the mind?*

This one simple practice helps you begin to build a framework based on the reality of the signs and signals being delivered, as opposed to the fears, worries and the Internet searches the mind just can't keep from doing. Let yourself begin wherever you are, while holding judgment, anxieties, obsessions and fears at bay as best as you can. You might even say to this part of your mind, *Not right now. Right now it's the body's turn to speak.*

Once you get comfortable with a simple check-in like this, you can take it deeper by finding longer times, maybe upon awakening or before falling asleep, where you tune into something going on in your body in a deeper way. For instance, you could place a hand where the sensation is (if you can't reach it, put your focus there) and wonder to yourself, *"What are you trying to say to me?"* Be wide open to words, sensations, images, memories and any overall feelings. Give yourself the freedom of knowing you cannot do this wrong.

The Well of Healing Runs Deep

Years ago I wound up with a terrible rash that covered about three-quarters of my body. The fact that it was unsightly was the least of my worries. The real difficulty was that it itched intensely, especially at night. I had no idea how I got it or what to do about it. I couldn't find relief anywhere.

I suffered for months on end, waking up in the middle of the night feeling frazzled and broken. I saw every manner of healer; an acupuncturist, energy healer, a well-known dermatologist, a medicine man, my primary care physician, an ER doctor and more. I looked at my diet, my emotions and my past lives. On and on it went, but nothing seemed to help. The rash came and went as if it had a mind of its own; a sick, twisted, unknowable mind.

For years my acupuncturist had been telling me that in any healing journey you have to dig your well deep enough to find what you're looking for. He explained that most conditions will resolve themselves with the assistance of any approach, and that what mattered most was my willingness to stick with something long enough for it to be helpful.

He equated the healing journey to digging a well looking for water. He told me that if I kept digging a little and then changing spots, I was going to miss what I was looking for and wind up with a bunch of half-dug wells. *As in, no results.*

Ironically, that brings me to the other thing he kept telling me, that I needed more water. But it took me years for this truth to kick in. I thought it had to be more complicated than that. How could the solution just be more water? Water seemed anticlimactic somehow. Far too simple, common and obvious to be of use. I mean, *really*, what was happening to me was epic! It had to require some intense, complex and maybe even expensive and difficult to come by cure or procedure. Right?

Wrong!

During the times when I was not so patiently 'digging my well,' and before I had dug it deep enough to find the simple solution of water, *I learned how to take care of myself.* Believe me, this was no small thing. This alone was worth the price of all those sleepless nights and solutions-chasing madness.

More than that, it speaks to a truism in healing. In your attempts to learn from the body, the symptoms may not abate in the time you would like, giving you plenty of time to learn some deep and important things about yourself. That's why, no matter what's happening, learning the language of your body must be done with the greatest of patience, kindness and understanding.

I learned many lessons about caring for myself in the presence of something that was not going away. When the rash would flare up, I would drop all hope of a cure, all expectations of what should and should not be, and I would just be with myself. Like being with a baby I could not soothe, I held myself as lovingly as I could. I placed no conditions on me or my skin. Instead of resisting the rash, I learned how to practice radical self-care. More than anything else, this amounted to me being easier on myself inside my own mind.

I took baths to soothe my raw flesh and my battered and my broken spirit. I stopped seeking miracle cures and let go of the idea that my healing needed to be complicated and external. I gave in. I surrendered. Slowly, I got better. In fits and starts at first. And then in whole wonderful clumps.

After several years of this, I arrived at what I consider to be some guiding truths. Real healing requires patience and love. *Lots of it!* Underneath that, you have to make certain that the body's most basic biological and non-negotiable needs are met. At which point, you turn it all over to Something Greater than yourself and begin to see that beyond the language of the body is the movement and mysteries of the soul and the body coming together to help us grow in ways we could not, and would not, all on our own.

There will be times in all of our lives when no matter what we do, we will not get the 'results' we want in our body. This is to be expected. It doesn't mean that you're doing something wrong or being punished. It just means that some things take a long, *long* time to heal and some things may never heal in the way we want. But that no matter what, if you can see it all as teaching you something, you will heal and be made whole, bringing you closer to something you didn't even know you had gotten far away from to begin with.

When it seems like there's 'nothing' you can do, make a choice to intentionally step beyond being 'wrong' or 'broken' and into loving and forgiving yourself *without question*. Like the fiercest mama bear that ever lived, protect yourself (even if that means from yourself) from any words or beliefs that would undermine the truth. That being, that you are doing the very best that you can, *and so is your body.*

In the end, and even in the most difficult of experiences, there is magic and mystery on The Embodied Journey that will take you to places you would never have chosen on your own, but that if you can learn to stay close to yourself *through it all*, you may just find that the unknown destination you arrive at was far more than you could have ever asked for.

On Fixing & Seeking Guarantees

This is as good a time as any to talk about trying to fix ourselves or looking for guaranteed outcomes. Attempting to fix anything assumes it is broken. If we approach ourselves as broken and in need of fixing, it extends beyond the body and touches the heart and soul of who we believe ourselves to be. The resulting belief being, *there is something wrong with me.* I am broken, unloveable, wrong, fill in the blank. It is beyond painful to believe that there is something wrong with us and yet, it is how many of us feel a lot of the time. Sometimes, without even consciously knowing it.

This experience of 'wrongness' gets magnified when the body is not well or behaving in the way we want it to.

While there is nothing wrong with wanting painful things to go away, 'fixing' becomes problematic because it originates from a need to make difficult things go away. There's no room to simply be with what is in the spirit of discovering what it's all about. Being willing to see and be with what is there is a key ingredient in learning the language of the body.

But this won't be available to you when you are seeking a fix. I experienced this once when a practitioner asked me if I could receive the very thing I was trying to get away from. I thought my mind would explode with rage at the question. *What? No! Are you out of your mind? What are you talking about? Why would you say that to me? Why would I want to receive something I did not want? What a weird and disturbing thing to say to someone!*

Yet, what a profound and truthful question to pose. I now know why she said it. She wondered how close to the reality of my situation I could get without balking or denying what was there. Without bypassing the realities I could not admit to. Without looking for a quick outside fix.

A willingness to receive what we do not want while finding a new way to be with whatever is happening with our health, *maybe even making good use of it*, is a big part of being alive in a body in a trustworthy and satisfying way. This is vastly different from believing that something is wrong that needs to be avoided. Or fixed.

Which brings us to the risks and conditions of being alive in a body that offers no guarantees. We don't have full control over what will happen to us. Even though we know this, we still fight for it not to be so. We create lives, individually and collectively, that defy reality as we pretend we are in more control than we are. In turn, we seek experts who can offer us a guarantee. Not only is this an illusion, it leaves us separate from, and afraid of our own bodies because we refuse to be with the uncertainties and the uncontrollables of life.

To temper this, a question I often ask myself is, *Can I surrender to what my body is doing and become the one who embraces it all?* Not because I want it, like it, or hope what I do not want sticks around. But because I have come to see that until I can fully and completely say 'yes' to what is happening, I cannot choose what to do for my health and well-being from a clear and balanced place. Nor can I accept myself. *Or anyone else, for that matter.* Nor can I appreciate, and be with Life, on Life's terms.

One of the things that we can absolutely be guaranteed of as human beings is that discomfort is part of the experience of being alive. Regularly. Daily. Moment to moment, there is a good chance that something just won't feel right. Maybe it will be sensations of hunger or thirst. The need to eliminate. Temperature changes. Emotional ups and downs. Fatigue. Physical or mental pain. Illness. Tension. On and on it goes.

It's only natural to want to try and control what is happening to us by getting away from what doesn't feel good or by denying the realities that feel too big for us. Likely for as long as we have been around as a species, we have tried to come up with ways to alleviate experiences in life that feel too uncomfortable for us to be with. While our attempts to bring more ease, control and guaranteed outcomes to the experience of being alive have led to life-soothing remedies like painkillers, sleeping pills or sedatives, making whatever is bothering us go away, *comes at a cost.*

The cost can be that we often don't have the slightest idea of what is truly causing us to suffer. We can't see the root of our struggle. Instead of looking more deeply, we reach for the closest fix or a guarantee as delivered by another. All of it being the equivalent of shaking an angry fist at the storm that just flooded your basement, as opposed to recognizing that you have no control over the weather. And then doing what needs doing to shore your basement up.

To be clear, this is not a call to embrace martyrdom. Instead, it is a call to practice welcoming the Truth of Life, including the things we do not want, but that happen nonetheless. For no matter how much we think we can manage, no matter how crafty, skilled, rich, resourceful or creative we might be, there is no fixing or getting rid of everything that makes us uncomfortable. To try is a lie, and it is to refuse what it means to be in a human body.

YOUR OWN PERSONAL MEDICINE

I had the good fortune of working with a homeopath all through my children's childhood and beyond. One of her greatest suggestions was to keep a health journal on the kids. I would make note of how and when they got sick, what else was happening in their lives, what helped and what didn't. Over time, patterns began to emerge that I could identify, work with and even anticipate.

Equipped with these observations, I could predict how things would go before they ever took hold, which treatments were most effective and eventually, the approaches that would strengthen the systems that habitually went out of balance for them.

After a time, I began keeping a journal on myself, which now includes multiple versions because I have found it so powerful in understanding myself. These 'provings' as I refer to them, serve as the basis of my own Personal Medicine. 'Personal,' as in pertaining to a particular person, me. 'Medicine' as in the art and science of preserving and restoring my own health.

The volumes I have are made up of observations, wonderings, connections, approaches, feedback from practitioners, inspiration, information and more. It is unique to me and offers a meaningful and effective way to approach health in a time when conventional medicine is top heavy with bureaucrats, overburdened with red tape and chains of command and ineffective in its ability to get to the root causes of illness and suffering.

To care for yourself in this way is another one of those massive paradigm leaps because of the way that it places the responsibility of your body in your hands. Being accountable to the parts of your health that are within your power to control as you map out the particulars of you, what makes you sick and what you need to heal is at the heart of this powerful approach.

Choose a dedicated journal, three-ring binder or folder (I use all three) and just start. This is yours and you can do it any way that makes sense to you. Jot down symptoms, how you get sick, any connections you make, what is happening in your life, what you try, what works, what doesn't.

Give yourself time. Your observations may not make sense at first. You will encounter fears, limiting beliefs, conditioning and cultural messaging that keeps you stuck in anxious online searches and worst-case scenarios. But with consistent effort and curiosity, eventually you will find a way to move beyond your fears and into a greater fluency with the language of your body.

What if the things you most avoid about your body are important information?
Maybe even a blessing in disguise?

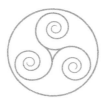

Obstacles

"The obstacle is the path."

- Zen expression

It is a sacred endeavor to learn how to be in your body while figuring out how to trust it. A big part of this journey includes being with what takes you *away* from your embodiment. There are so many things that can get in the way of a loving and satisfying relationship with your body. Obstacles like judgment, distractions, quick fix mindsets, expert-seeking, habits, fears and more that can get in the way of you fully inhabiting yourself.

It's not easy being in a body. There are so many sensations, pressures, thoughts, beliefs and experiences that go along with how we feel about our bodies and what it means to inhabit them. That's why it can feel preferable to leave them or let someone else be in charge of them.

Unfortunately, it has become a widely accepted way of 'living' to leave our bodies and what it is we are experiencing.

Take my college students and how they 'party.' The way they use drugs, alcohol and casual sex to knock down the stress. To keep from feeling what they don't want to feel. Using substances and superficial experiences of intimacy to take them away from what feels too hard to be with. That being, *the experience of being in a body.*

I know this place. *All too well.* It was how I lived for years. Partying, eating and exercising to excess and as punishment. Self-loathing and worthlessness arising out of the choices I was making. It was only when I began to feel how horrible what I was doing to myself felt that I could shift. Only when I was willing to encounter the obstacles to good and fulfilling connection with my body did things, *slowly and steadily*, begin to change.

While incredibly difficult, excruciating even, to come up against what was keeping me from myself, it was real. And it was true. *Obstacles are an absolutely unavoidable part of The Embodied Journey.* So that's where I began. Not because I knew what I was doing initially, *and certainly not because I liked it*, but because the obstacles loomed so large, I just had to address them. There was no way forward except straight through what I had been avoiding and deceiving myself about.

Wires Crossed

Without addressing the obstacles that stand between us and our bodies, we are doomed to keep repeating what doesn't work, feel good or honor the preciousness of our own lives.

This approach is not so obvious in the world we live in. There is a strong current in our culture that tells us to get away from what feels bad, and we have seemingly endless options now for medicating our bodies against what doesn't feel good. That's why addressing what is getting in the way does not occur to many of us as a viable option.

As mammals, we're wired to get away from what causes pain, so it's only natural to move away from what we don't want or like. But when we cross-pollinate this basic instinct with a culture that makes it so easy to disconnect from ourselves with distractions, drugs and workaholism, we have a perfect storm for leaving our bodies in ways that are detrimental to us, as well as those around us.

Our modern-day existence, with all of its ways to medicate ourselves, exploits our built-in survival systems.

Getting away from what hurts us is a necessary survival and coping mechanism. This self-preservation instinct keeps us alive and out of harm's way. This instinct shows up in something as straightforward as the way you would pull your hand away from fire, remove a splinter from your foot or get away from harsh external elements like the cold, the wind or severe heat.

However, in modern day life, many of our pains are self- and culturally-induced, with no connection whatsoever to imminent survival requirements. We see this when our chronically stressed minds, stuck in survival mode, see traffic, our daily schedules, getting the promotion we want or our kids getting into the school we want, as matters of life or death.

This is where our wires have gotten crossed when it comes to what is harmful. In other words, because our nervous systems are so chronically on alert, our dangers have been exaggerated and even made up in our own minds. Driven by high states of alarm and overwhelm, it is only natural to want to try and get away from so much of our lives. But this has left us deeply confused about what to avoid and what to deal with. *A basic, primal instinct to avoid harm has been flipped on its head, and is now bringing suffering and the need to medicate ourselves rather than seeking true relief.*

We're told, *take this edible, binge watch this series, spend hours scrolling to get away from feeling what you're feeling.* I recognize that being told to deal with what you typically avoid in order to come more completely into your body can sound too contrary to the current narrative. Can feel too painful. Or like too much effort. But if we don't notice the ways we put up obstacles to our full embodiment, we'll miss out on some of the most important information we will ever receive. Information crucial to our ability to navigate the world. Information that lets us know what it is to be alive. *Not to mention that covering up the pain of living doesn't make it go away, and acting as if something is not there, only makes it worse.*

You'll know exactly what I mean if you've ever avoided paying attention to a health issue early on, only for it to blow up and become much worse of a problem later on. We can also see this happening all around us in the epidemics of obesity, stress, chronic lifestyle-related diseases, addiction and more; all of the imbalances in living we as a culture are dealing with and that are based in part, on avoidance. And disconnection. And the wrong things being used as 'solutions.' As well as an overall denial of the root causes of our suffering.

But if we can allow ourselves to be with what keeps us from establishing a healthy embodiment, we open ourselves to the possibility of being with our bodies in a new way. Ways that have nothing to do with ignoring anything, but instead are about honing our attention and focus when something isn't working and using that as guidance. An agreement we make with ourselves to notice when something just doesn't feel right and using that as an opportunity to learn more about what makes us tick.

Right about now, you might be thinking, *it's easier to not know. It's easier to not feel what's there.* I completely understand if what I'm proposing sounds like too much work, scary even, to consider being with what you usually try to get away from. This response is to be expected if this is a new way of thinking for you. But whether or not you're in your body, whether you're willing to accept what is there or not, *what is there is there.* And any obstacles you engage with to keep you from knowing that, *are just that.* Obstacles.

Bottom line? If you've built a relationship with your body based on avoidance, you won't know what you need or what your body is telling you. *And you certainly won't be able to trust a body you avoid.*

But if you're in your body, choosing to be with the 'obstacles' from the perspective that they carry the codes to take you back to yourself, you will have tapped into body-based wisdom which can serve as the gold standard for where you need to put your attention.

And, you can ultimately take those obstacles and transform them into golden opportunities for living well.

Demons or Goddesses? You Decide

There are some Eastern traditions, Yoga being one of them, where it is understood that the obstacles in our lives symbolize demons plaguing us. Demons from this point of view being anything that we would say hurts us. As the mythologies go, if we can learn the name of the demon, it will transform itself into a goddess and bless us.

Nothing captures the power of learning to face our obstacles like this perspective. If you can see that there is value in moving towards what you typically avoid, the blessings will be numerous and far-reaching. Beyond even what you can imagine from where you currently stand.

For the sake of argument, *what if it were true? What if the things you most avoid about your body are important information?* Maybe even a blessing in disguise?

As you can see, there's a lot to contemplate here when it comes to what keeps you from having a sound and trusting relationship with your body. Uncovering what gets in the way will take time. Uncovering the obstacles will ask that you be good to yourself as you explore. This is a lifelong process of getting to know yourself, and just like the proverbial onion, you keep peeling back layer after layer, discovering new obstacles, *as well as potential goddesses*, as you go.

Common Obstacles

Let's take time now to look at some of the most common obstacles that separate us from our bodies and what they need. While there are many, I've found the following to be particularly powerful in their capacity to either be a demon or a goddess. They are:

- Judgment
- Distractions
- Quick Fix Mentality & Expert Seeking
- Habits
- Fear

The following pages offer you an opportunity to hold yourself to a code of taking personal responsibility, while allowing yourself to begin wherever you are as you explore these common obstacles. Take all the time you need while giving yourself lots of kindness and understanding along the way. You have legitimate reasons for where you are right now and for doing what you do. Kindly include your reasons, while making a commitment to meet up with what stops you in the spirit of being blessed by what you discover.

The Harsh Voice of Judgment

No one, I repeat *no one*, will be harder on you and your body *than you*. But here's the truth, no baby comes into the world judging their unique bodily experience. Any of the ways that we have learned to be hard on ourselves was never ours to begin with. External judgements were laid on us by those around us; born of their own troubles with being in a body in a sacred way.

Before we ever learned the language of judgment, we were just *being* in our bodies. In our early days and years of life, *we were our bodies!* There was no mind separate from our physical selves. We were just one, unified human. No judgment. No criticism. Just us in a body, living and having experiences. Some pleasant, some painful. Some pretty, some messy.

Back then, our physical appearance meant nothing about us. Chubby thighs? *Perfect*. Belly rolls? *Adorable*. Bald? *Not even thinking about it*. If you have seen the pure joy of a young child with no self-consciousness about their body, you have seen Life at its vibrant best.

As a mother of young children, watching my two kids run naked through our house, completely at home in their own bodies, moved me beyond words. How I yearned to feel that freedom again within my own body. It was so liberating and healing to watch them run through the house calling out, *"Naked night!"* It mattered not who was around, or what the schedule might call for. The joy and aliveness of their bodies had to be expressed. *Fully unbridled.* In these moments, not a single criticism blocked them from their natural expression and full embodiment.

How can we possibly know the authentic fullness of who we are, including all the gifts of being in a body, while we're condemning it? Judgment separates us from ourselves as we compare and judge our various bodily parts, worried about what others are thinking and decide we are less than valuable based on what we see in the mirror. But if you can ease up on the self-judgment, you begin to find your way into a satisfying and connected experience with your body.

Lest you think judgment and criticism is the best way to motivate yourself, *think again.* Judgment erodes trust within and without. It is a cruel taskmaster that deadens the vital relationship with not only ourselves, but all of Life. Judging your body shuts down the possibility of discovering important pieces of information that could prove invaluable to navigating life in your body. Most of all, *to judge is to condemn,* and maybe even hate, our very own selves. To judge ourselves is to find ourselves unworthy, with worthlessness being about the most painful of all the human experiences.

If you cannot accept your body and what it is worth, you will not value it. We do not protect what we do not value. *What we do not value, we do not care for.* Neglected and unprotected, we abandon the necessary boundaries and actions required to healthfully move through a world filled with far too many life-depleting and body-denying choices.

BEYOND JUDGMENT

If I weren't judging what was happening right now in my body, what would I see? What would I know?

This is a powerful question to ponder with a wide-open mind and heart. This is not an opportunity to be hard on yourself, or to find the definitive answer. Instead, think of it like a Zen puzzle for your mind that works on you over time. Be as light as a cloud while you let this question float within you, watching what happens when you suspend judgment. This isn't something you can figure out with hard work, mental concentration and a furrowed brow. Instead, it is a kind of revealing that makes itself available to you when you clear the obstruction of judgment.

If we are to experience embodiment as an alive, informative and pleasurable journey, we must transcend the judge and jury of the mind. We must be willing to go beyond our ideas of right and wrong, while suspending our pursuit of perfection. Otherwise, we are left only to condemn our very existence.

Each and every day, what would I see, what would I know, if I wasn't making myself or my body wrong?

Distractions

There's no doubt that we're living with more distractions in our lives than ever before. Cell phones, video games, busy work schedules, sports and leisure commitments, social media, streaming services, intoxicants, must-see videos, apps and more. The distractions block us from being in a body, feeling all that is there. Running from one thing to the next, we distract ourselves right out of ourselves and somehow, *still call it living*. Still believe that this is the very best life has to offer us.

But there's an enormous cost to prioritizing things that have nothing to do with keeping us healthy and satisfied in the truest sense of those words. Choosing the feeling of being numb over the feeling of being alive, our capacity to nourish ourselves diminishes as we avoid facing the natural challenges of life in a body. Distractions are the sugar coating on a pill we believe is too hard to swallow. That pill being what it means to be human, and what it takes to be alive and care for our body in a sacred way.

Maybe distractions feel good momentarily. Eventually though, we no longer know how to be quiet or how to slow down enough to be at home in our own bodies. And because so many of us are so caught up in the distractions, we don't see how it's actually not working for any of us because we've come to believe that it's 'normal' now to live like this.

In a world flooded with easy, cheap and accessible distractions, we forget how to be alone or how to listen. Regularly stressed, in pain, unable to focus, overwhelmed and pushed to the edge, it just feels better to get out of ourselves any way we can. The frenetic pace of our lives, the technological obsessions, the compulsive buying, the staying busy at any cost, the seemingly endless ways of medicating ourselves while being more interested in following other people than living our own lives, is disconnecting us from the very ground of existence itself. Our bodies.

When we choose to distract ourselves, *nothing actually changes.* Not only are the difficulties still there, we now have a blindness to their existence. Now we are not dealing with the reality of our lives, nor are we developing the skills we need and would develop if we were meeting the challenges of being in a body in an intentional and focused way. All we've done is put distance between us and our body. This may be an okay short-term strategy, but building a life on distraction erodes our capacity to trust ourselves, and diminishes our ability to rely on our body as a guidance system for navigating the world. Living a distracted life means problems go unnoticed for far too long, right up to the point when they become a crisis.

What are we all trying to get away from?

What are we avoiding?

Facing these questions can stir up a range of emotions, from overwhelm and pain, to anxiety and grief. Perhaps this is why we often banish them to the basement of our awareness; uncertain we want to admit or see why we are so intent on distracting ourselves.

I once heard someone say, *"Your attention is your most precious resource. Guard it well."* This is another one of those great leaps forward. The leap being to guard where you place your attention, and in whose hands you put it.

Staying Human

Let's pause here to highlight the biggest of the outward distractions; being in front of a screen. The ways that many of us are using the technologies is one of the surest ways to distract ourselves right out of our own bodies and therefore, *our very lives*. The undeniable seduction of the devices separates us from what the body is experiencing and needing. Somehow, we don't notice the achy back, the sore neck, the strained eyes, the fact we are ignoring a bathroom urge or that we're exhausted and need to sleep.

We miss the look on a loved one's face or the tone of their voice. We miss the changing of the Earth's seasons and her daily offerings. The pull of what comes across a screen is so powerful that it makes us forget what is most important to us, and is strong enough to make us overlook or deny what it is to be human. *Especially when it comes to the body and what it needs, there is no competing with what comes across a screen.*

If we have any hope of navigating the technologies while still staying human, we must put our bodies first whenever we are in front of a screen. *Get in the habit of giving priority to your body.* Build in specific moments to tend to the needs of your embodiment. Get up. Move around. Get food (off screen). Step outside. Call instead of texting or emailing. Talk to someone face to face.

Keep connected to your body and what it means to be human at all times when using the technologies. Place beautiful objects around your computer. Set yourself up so you can look out a window. Put stickers on your phone to remind you of what is most important to you. A former student of mine posted a sticky note on the back of her phone with the question, *"Why am I here?"* It was her way of taking a beat before obsessively checking her phone. It also speaks to the greatest question any human being can ever ask of themselves: WHY AM I HERE?

Is your greatest and highest calling and expression to be at the beck and call of a machine? Or is it something more? The incessant call of a machine may be one of the biggest impediments to satisfying embodiment. The slow and subtle ways of the body, along with the needs that must be regularly tended to, cannot compete with the speed, the noise and the 24/7 nature of what comes across a screen.

Life with the devices has trained us towards acceleration, convenience and instant gratification. All of which are the enemies of the body. Instead of succumbing to what will never satisfy you in the way you are needing it to, let your own body be your true North Star when it comes to how you live your life. Not a bunch of wires and chips.

The Quick Fix Mentality & Expert-Seeking

These two obstacles go hand in hand and are deeply ingrained in the culture at large. Many of us have become increasingly more comfortable looking to sources outside of ourselves to tell us what to feel, what to put in our bodies and how to behave. These same sources propagate the myth that taking care of ourselves should be quick, easy and someone else's job.

This is shaky footing when it comes to our health and well-being. If we were paying close attention, we would see how quick fixes rarely live up to the guarantee of what is being offered. Believing in them to the exclusion of the real truths of the body, steals our agency and keeps us infantalized and subservient to something outside of us. This is a major obstacle to finding our own way to health and well-being. Not to mention self-trust.

Which takes us to another issue with quick fixes and expert-seeking. Many of us blame ourselves when the outside fixes don't work or when the advice of the experts fails us. Now we are even more doubtful and suspicious of our bodies. But what if the reason this kind of externalized approach doesn't work is because it's not aligned with what we most need? Or isn't honest about its claims? Being in a body is a life*long* (as in, *not quick*) relationship with yourself that must be cultivated and honored over time. Especially when the body does not feel well.

Am I suggesting you don't seek outside opinions or external remedies? *Absolutely not.* What I am suggesting is that we do so from a place of personal responsibility and sovereignty, rather than a child-like state of mind that believes someone else can magically make our boo-boos go away. Used consciously and conscientiously, pills, procedures and outside support can be helpful and life-saving. But we know all too well that relying exclusively on these approaches can have troubling side effects. Worse yet, focusing on quick fixes and expert advice above our own participation takes what we don't want to look at and sweeps it under the rug. Hidden there, we never learn the necessary truths that could lead us to fuller health and well-being.

Breaking Up With Bad Habits

We all have them. Habits of thinking, eating, moving, feeling and relating. Like a well-worn path, they offer familiar comfort and a sense of security in the world. They give us something to count on and lean into, serving as an oasis of stability in an ever-changing and unpredictable world.

Yet, as much as habits can support us, *they can also limit us.* The habits we cling to unconsciously keep us from our goals, dreams, desires. So even though our habits may be keeping us from a good relationship with our bodies, we choose them anyway because they are the devil we know and prefer. Over time, we continue choosing life-depleting habits, even when we are well aware that they're not working, and maybe even harming us. Like the foods we continue to eat even though we know they're making us ill, sluggish or causing us to break out.

One of the most energizing things you can do with ingrained habits is look at what it costs you to be doing what you do. Imagine if you could add up all of the habits you keep and the equation would show you a visual depicting the life that you have chosen. *What would your image be?* While potentially startling, this is not a bad way to think about the behaviors we engage in every single day. As in, what are we doing regularly without realizing what it's costing us?

More to the point, what habits serve to support a good relationship with your body and which ones get in the way? Check in with yourself regularly asking, *Is this really working for me?*

Observe yourself. Be willing to change things up in how you eat, move and how much time you spend in front of a screen. Be willing to refrain, every once in a while, from what you always do. That might mean taking something out of your diet now and again, adding something in or switching out a soda for water. It could mean not looking at your phone first thing in the morning or not watching a show just before bedtime.

There's no doubt that habits have an important role to play in our lives. They help us to not have to reinvent the wheel each day, which leaves us with energy we can use for other things. But they become an obstacle when the automatic nature of these behaviors does not allow us to notice what is no longer working. Breaking up with habits that no longer serve you helps you to get closer to living in a body you feel good being in.

Fear of Change

Deep down, we all know that when we begin to change our relationship to our bodies, our lives will change everywhere else. That knowing sparks fear. *But why?* Don't we want things to be different? Yes, but only if certain things remain the same. We want to lose weight, trust ourselves more or feel better, *while leaving the rest of our lives untouched.*

Part of us says, *Come on, we've made it this far, we're still alive, why rock the boat? Why risk the unknown? Who knows what will happen? Maybe it won't feel good, or be safe. Maybe people won't like us anymore. Maybe we won't fit in, or god forbid, have to let go of something we don't want to lose!*

Acknowledging this push and pull within ourselves is essential because parts of us will *always* fear things being different. *This is to be expected.* But if we don't acknowledge the fact that part of us wants in, and part of us doesn't, we will always be at odds with ourselves. More to the point, we will sabotage our efforts, under-cutting our attempts at making change. To help smooth this out, we need to admit that change has a big power behind it.

That big power being its wild card nature to change you in ways you never expected. You can never be quite sure what part of your life will be touched, swept away or no longer fit. Make no mistake about it, change is a dis-ruptive force. It brings with it both gain and loss. Which is precisely why we resist. We want to be in charge and have some kind of guarantee that things will change, but only exactly as we want them to. *And no more.* We want to be able to put that genie back into the bottle at a moment's notice. But we all know how that turns out. Once the genie is out, *it's out.*

That's why despite how challenged we can be in our bodies, despite how much we know something has to give, *we still resist.* We struggle with that big unknowable unknown. So even though we might give our standard explanation of being too busy, not knowing how to start, not feeling we are worth it, these can be just symptoms of a far greater fear of the unknown and stirring up all of its wild nature.

What will happen to my life if I start feeling and looking better?

How will I socialize if I no longer do things that don't feel good in my body?

How will I connect with others when I make new choices different from what they are familiar or comfortable with?

Fear is not an obstacle to be ignored, bypassed or underestimated. Fear alone can sabotage anything you're trying to do if you do not honor and include it. For despite what it feels like now to be in your body, welcome or not, *it's what you know.* It's what's familiar, and how you know yourself. This is also how everyone around you knows you. Your present reality feels safe, even if it's uncomfortable or painful.

FEAR AS GOD

In ancient yogic teachings, fear was seen as a potent motivator. Fear being considered the most powerful of the body's primal energies that also includes anger and lust. Fear is directly connected to our animal nature and is beyond the rational mind. If you have ever had a health scare for yourself or someone close to you, you know the powerful motivating force fear has to make us change, *when we otherwise wouldn't.*

That's why, to intentionally work with fear when we are not necessarily in a crisis can be a powerful way back to the health and well-being we all seek. To use fear consciously as a way to break through a mind that likes to deny what it does not want to know.

A perspective I often come back to is imagining that fear and God are one and the same. In Sanskrit, there is a word that is both a name for fear and one of the names for God. This understanding implies that if you can be with fear, the most charged of the animal energies, *while observing it*, the power will take you directly back to God. That's how powerful it is!

But don't take my word for it. Try it. Begin to imagine what you're afraid of. Instead of trying to get away from it, what if you saw it as a direct route to God? In our attempts to manage all the unknowns in our lives, isn't fear exactly what keeps us from knowing the face of God that makes the most sense to us?

To embrace our fears is to know ourselves. And to know ourselves is to know God.

In the end, to know ourselves is to encounter all the obstacles that prevent us from being at home in our bodies. The more you can see this as a natural unfolding and unwinding, the more you can align with Something Greater than just yourself. And the more you can do this, the more those demons will be transmuted into goddesses, who will then turn around and bless your Embodied Journey.

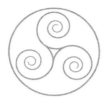

You Must Be Willing to Break From a Sick Herd

"It is no sign of health to be well adapted to a profoundly sick society."

- J. Krishnamurti

As human beings, we are both human and mammal. As such, we're wired to stay within the protection and the comfort of the herd. To seek security and guidance from those around us. *But what happens when the herd is sick?* What are we to do when the culture around us is condoning ways of living that make us stressed, ill and imbalanced in order to belong? And how are we to stay true to trusting our bodies when the herd, and what it is pulling for, is sick?

A few years ago, I was away in New York City for a movement workshop. Every day we went through a combination of movement experiences that we sometimes did on our own, and sometimes came into physical contact with others. During one of the last exercises of the weekend, they partnered me with someone I instantly knew, *I did not want to touch or be touched by.*

Instinctively, my body gave a clear and resounding message of revulsion. This did not happen on the thinking level, as in *This guy is gross or creepy*, but at the bodily level, where waves of unease and disgust washed over me, again and again. There was no denying how I felt. Yet a lifetime of social conditioning rose up to challenge my body-based knowing. My herd-oriented mind began to scramble. I couldn't reconcile what I needed to do for myself in that moment with what I imagined 'they' were expecting of me.

Despite the clarity in my body, my mind was screaming, *What will this look like to everyone in the room if you refuse to partner with him? They'll think this is my fault. That I'm being hysterical! Overly sensitive! Problematic! They'll take his side. They'll turn against me. You'll look like an idiot. This is all your fault. Why can't you just suck it up?*

My herd mind mentality was freaking out, and the message was loud and clear: *Do not buck the system.* Do not step outside what the group is expecting of you. *Or else.*

But what about me? Every thought racing through my mind was at war with my body-based guidance. My body was not at all confused. *It was absolutely and undeniably repulsed.* But the part of me tethered to the group mind would not, could not, let that be. Honoring my body's wisdom would mean risking upsetting the herd, and what was expected of me.

So even though a piece of deep, primal information from my body kept saying, *Don't do it. Do not partner with him*, my socially-oriented mind would not budge. It felt too risky when I looked at it through their eyes and I could not get past the terror that I would be publicly humiliated. I was left with what felt like an impossible choice: *Honor the signals of my body and risk social condemnation, or give in to what was expected of me and dishonor myself.*

What did I do? I wish I could say that I chose for myself, *but I did not.* Unable to resolve the deep divide between taking care of myself and the social demands as I anticipated them, I shut down; frozen by the irreconcilable predicament I found myself in, I literally cannot even remember what happened. I must have gone through the motions of the exercise, but because I was so shut down, I have no conscious recollection of what actually happened.

This moment captures the deep-seated and primal fears in all of us around whether or not we have a right to honor our needs and inner knowings, *and still belong.* My experience speaks directly to the inherent struggle between trusting and caring for the self and our non-negotiable survival drive to belong. This drive is a basic, instinctual, often unconscious need that underlies our individual actions and is the physiological glue for keeping communities intact.

But it also sets up the classic dilemma between the needs of the individual and the requirements of belonging. The very same dilemma that can leave us unsure about whether or not we have a right to personal needs that may be different from what the group expects. *Or demands.* Struggling under the social expectations and conditioning that tells us what we need to do to fit in, can leave us wondering what will happen to us if we choose differently.

Survival & Belonging

This social drive to belong is so strong, we may choose to do things to be loved and accepted by others that are in direct conflict to what we need or to what we know. Our survival drive for belonging is so great, we will sacrifice ourselves and our well-being to remain in the good graces of others. *No. Matter. What.* Even if it dishonors who we are, what we are experiencing and what we most need.

While there is an essential survival imperative for us to subjugate our individual needs to the needs of the group, what happens when the social requirements, *spoken or not*, are out of alignment with real, human biological needs and drives? Worse yet, what happens when the herd is expecting us to do something that in actuality brings us harm? And what recourse do we have when the sickness in the herd has become the expectation, *even the non-negotiable requirement*, for how we must live? *As in, do what the rest of us are doing, or else...*

Coupled with the built-in mammalian survival drive to belong, each of us has a lifetime of experiences and messaging from our families, friends, school systems, workplaces, media and health institutions about what we must do in order to belong. Beliefs about how we must show up, what is acceptable and what is not 'allowed' when it comes to our body and its behaviors. Some of this is benign and well-intentioned. Some of it is ignorant, destructive and driven by agendas that have nothing to do with what a body most needs.

The tricky thing is, what we feel we must do to belong is so ingrained in us that for the most part, *we never even question it.* It just feels like this is how it is. *This is how it must be.* It's the equivalent of asking a fish, *How's the water?* We're so inseparable from the sea of social conditioning ingrained in us that we don't even recognize the waters we're swimming in. Never mind that we even have a choice.

Because of our deep and primal survival need to belong to one another, we can live blind to all the ways that modern life is training us away from the basic biological truths and necessities of our very own bodies. Through the confusing, misleading and often erroneous information we receive from the advertising world, we convince ourselves of the wrong things in order to fit in with others. And because so many of us have agreed to some very detrimental ways of treating our bodies, it's easy to believe that what we're doing is normal because of how many of us are doing it.

I think somewhere down deep we all know how devastating this is. Equally, it seems insurmountable. Like it would be too much of a risk to break free from what is happening all around us. Too much to break free from the herd. So we stay.

It is deeply wired into us to stay with the herd. *So deep we will even stay when it is making us sick, rather than to risk being ostracized for making different choices.* The core imperative? *Remain at all costs.* Even to your own detriment. Which is why when we notice how we might be abandoning our health and well-being by lining up with what others think, by how we were raised, by social media influencers or by the pressures to conform to what the marketers are selling us, we will absolutely encounter deep-seated, unconscious fears of abandonment, public humiliation and even attack when we consider choosing differently than those around us.

It is right at this point of having to decide between us and going along, *when all the alarms are going off*, that we have an opportunity. Each time we encounter an experience where *we are knowing and needing one thing*, and still desiring the promise of safety, belonging and acceptance, we are at the crossroads of a life-changing moment.

I can choose to stay with what I am experiencing and decide from there. Or I can choose to do what is expected of me, whether it works or not.

But of course, in order to even contemplate this, *you must be in your body*; willing to include everything, while taking responsibility for what you are experiencing as you navigate in real time, life in a body while in the company of others.

AWARE OF ME

Because so much of our social conditioning sits in our unconscious, we need ways to access it if we have any hope of distinguishing between what we need and what others expect of us. What I mean by this is we have spent decades learning what it takes for us to belong. That means it's not always so obvious that we have a choice in this regard.

For instance, *how often do you engage in unhealthy behaviors because that's what those around you are doing? How often do you abdicate responsibility for your health to an expert because that is the accepted paradigm in the culture, and to do anything else feels heretical?* As in, this is what others are doing, and so must I. This is what my doctor or public health campaign says I must do, *and so I must.*

To trust our bodies, what they need and what they are experiencing, requires that we remain sovereign unto our own experience in the presence of others. *This is incredibly difficult to do!*

We are built to take our cues from one another and to reference others to know how we're doing. This is solid survival behavior when you are referencing a healthy herd. But absolutely disastrous when not.

How can we tell the difference? *By being in our bodies and learning to listen to what they are saying to us, despite who's in front of us and what they expect us to do.* Not easy, but a powerful path to becoming a healthy and fully functioning member of the herd.

Try this. When you are with other people, get in the regular habit of saying to yourself, *I am aware of...*

Become aware of things in the environment like temperature and any specifics in your surroundings. For instance, *I am aware of... the warm sun, that beautiful flower, the look on her face, the table, the picture...*

Become aware of the thoughts and emotions you are experiencing. *I am aware of... feeling distant, excited, happy, stressed...*

Finally, become aware of your body. *I am aware of feeling hungry, tired, in pain, at ease...*

Let yourself circulate through what's outside of you to what's inside of you. Feel free to go in any order and to stay with any layer that feels particularly grounding or informative at any moment.

The entire point of this practice is to locate yourself in your own bodily experience whenever you are around other people. This helps you in two ways. It gets you anchored in the present moment, which means you will be less likely to choose from past hurts or future worries. And it trains you to know that you are your own unique person who may or may not need or want what the herd is currently offering.

But the only way any of this works is if you allow yourself to be where you are while seeing that everything you are noticing and experiencing is worthy of your attention and is valid information to make decisions from; whether others see it or not, agree with you or not.

A Leap of Faith

Being a mammal with a human mind is both an extraordinary and challenging experience. It is not easy to honor your membership in the group while also discerning what works for you and what does not. The power of conformity is that strong. Your need for belonging can drive you to go against your better judgment in order to feel accepted. Trapped in this struggle between what you need and the expectations of the group is never a comfortable place to be.

As a parent who made choices that were significantly different from how I was raised and how the culture in general was doing things around child-rearing, I felt that discomfort deeply. Getting sideways looks at family gatherings or from that parent or teacher at the kids' school, challenged me down to my very core. I grew up believing that if I didn't do it 'right' according to others, I would be banished. Kicked out. Shamed. So when I began making choices different from those around me, it pulled up all my fears around belonging and affiliation. I struggled terribly, and at times still do, with the fear that others might be offended, upset or threatened by the choices I make to care for my body.

But I have also experienced that when I am steeped in doing what is best for me, there is no dilemma. When I am fully committed to myself, to being in a body and giving it what it needs, I can be anywhere and with anyone. Or, I know how to give myself the permission I need to make a different choice if I determine that I am in the 'wrong' situation for me; having learned to get comfortable choosing not to be in places or spend time with people who do not make way for life-affirming needs.

Interestingly enough, it has been the most difficult experiences that have taught me the power the herd has over me; teaching me how often, and under what circumstances, I will betray the trust I have in myself. With each experience though, I learn more about what I believe I must do, or how I must compromise, in order to stay in connection with others. It has shown me the painful dilemma we all face regarding the choices we feel we must make between self-care and belonging.

As more time passes, I have come to value the challenging times with others because it has taught me so much about who I am, who I am not, what I need and what I do not need. All of this translates into the greatest offering I will ever make to the world; me as a balanced and healthy member who contributes to creating a balanced and healthy herd.

So whether others see it this way or not, I have come to know the value of a healthy individual as *the starting place* for building a healthy community. This is what motivates me to stay true to myself; trusting that there is always a place for me in the herd when I am my healthiest and most authentic self. Trusting that the very best thing I will ever offer to the world is to be as true to myself and what I need, as I can be.

A Selfless Act

While many of us have come to believe that caring for ourselves is a *selfish* act, what if the opposite was true? *What if you, being good to you, made you good to all of us?* What if, taking care of you, is the most SELFLESS act you will ever engage in, in your entire life?

How's this landing with you? This is a big one on The Embodied Journey of learning to trust yourself, so let's take a moment here to pause, for this is seminal to your ability to do right by your own life. *Pause. Pause. Pause.* It is also the royal road to self-trust and to you being a healthy contributing member of any community that you belong to. *Pause.* And yet, this is exactly the place where many, many of us get lost. *Do you know what I'm talking about? Pause.*

But what if it were true? What if it were true that it was actually selfish for you to not take care of yourself? Big, big pause.

I'll even go one further. *How could it be anything but true?* As a society, a community, a family, a team, the whole will only ever be as good as the sum total of all of the individuals who make up that group. *How could it be otherwise?* How could we possibly expect that a bunch of sick and imbalanced individuals will lead anywhere but to a sick herd?

This is another one of those absolutely monumental paradigm leaps. Many of us have developed entire personas based on being the one who is *never* selfish. Translation? Never tends to their own needs. Likely does not even know what they need. Unfortunately, those around us can actually like when we have no needs. Can like having those in our midst who don't require anything, and who only make way for us.

Because this has been so conditioned into us, and because the selfless among us reap so many rewards for being this person in the lives of others, the conscious mind will often not pick this one up until we are at our wits end. Until we are feeling burdened and put upon. Until it is glaringly obvious that we have neglected our needs in favor of fitting in. So the next time you find yourself feeling taken for granted, or like your needs are left unmet, use it as an opportunity to retrace and rework in your mind what it was about the experience that didn't work for you.

It is in these crucial moments of creating space for ourselves, even in hindsight, that we can catch a glimpse of what we need through the experience of *not getting what we needed.* It is in these spaces that we come to know ourselves and to find the courage that we need to be both sovereign unto our own experience, while still belonging. This is what our world most needs. More of us living as fully embodied sovereign individuals, contributing from wholeness.

This doesn't mean you won't encounter struggles with those who do not understand what you're doing when it comes to caring for yourself. It doesn't mean that when you start to change how you are in relationship with others that there won't be some friction to work out. What it does mean is that by staking your claim around your body and what it truly needs, you will grow in clarity and self-trust while learning to strengthen your resolve to care for yourself in a sacred way. Best of all, you learn how to be with others in a respectful way who are making different choices than you.

This is a lifelong practice that requires lots and lots of permission. Permission to be in your body and to act on what you are finding there. Permission to get stuck and to make mistakes. Permission to step beyond social expectations and demands. Most importantly, permission to decide for yourself what you will move towards or away from when it comes to your body. *No matter what it looks like to anyone else. Even if it looks selfish to either you or others.*

An Antidote to a Sick Herd

Hands down, learning how to trust your body and what it needs from the inside-out is the antidote to a sick herd. It will always be a healthy choice to break from a herd that has been unduly influenced by marketing campaigns, junk foods, choices, values and technology platforms that have nothing to do with what a real human being actually needs to thrive. You and your ability to tap into what your body needs is the antidote to the seductions and fears that have pulled too many of us away from being healthy together.

As hard as this might be to hear, *when the herd is sick, you must be willing to recognize that.* You must be willing to break from any expectations or behaviors that encourage or engender ill health and dis-ease. This does not mean that you leave everyone you know and love. But it does mean that you learn over time, through trial and error, not to reference, not to look to or agree to, what violates you and what you really need.

Otherwise, you are subject to go along with what is not working and what is broken, no matter what that does to all of us. By agreeing to the wrong things, you contribute to what is sickening us all. Even though we might believe that following what others are doing is a sensible way to fit in or an easy way to sidestep difficult moments, we are creating far more difficulty by our unwillingness to 'fit out,' when that would be the best choice for all.

Against the Grain

The air is cold and crisp. The sky is clear blue. New fallen snow sparkles everywhere. I'm where I most want to be; out on a run with the person (my husband) I most want to be with. Pure perfection. *Except for one tiny thing.* I feel like crap. My legs are heavy. My mood is murky. My motivation and energy level are barely enough to keep me going. *How did I get here?* By violating myself the night before because that's what I thought I needed to do to stay in connection with others.

It all started innocently enough when our neighbors came over for dinner bringing a home-made bottle of wine. At this point in my life, I rarely drink alcohol. But it seemed worth the experience to avoid looking ungrateful, so I accepted the most miniscule amount. The first few sips were great, but then I was done. Only some part of me would not let myself be done because no one else was. So I drank a few more sips, and that was all it took to leave me hungover the next morning.

I know it might sound ridiculous that a grown woman can only handle a few sips of alcohol, but that would be missing the point. The point being, alcohol mostly just doesn't work for me anymore. *And what really doesn't work for me is to override the signals I get from my body.*

I overrode what was right for me because it was what I thought I needed to do to stay in connection. I drank more than my body wanted because I did not want to hurt another person's feelings. If I'm being completely honest, I did it because I didn't want them to see me as a prude or a lightweight. I did it because part of me wasn't sure if I could still be part of the herd if what I needed for me was different from what they were choosing for themselves.

And there it is in a nutshell. While we say we do things because we do not want to hurt or offend, the truth is, we are terrified to be on the 'outs' with another. Scared to death to go against the grain, we sacrifice ourselves and our well-being at the altar of fitting in. Which brings me to what I have been exploring and wondering about for years.

Is there a way we can find our place in the world of other people, while still taking care of ourselves?

A place where we do not need to make apologies, give excuses, dumb down or hide who we are and what we need? Maybe even, *at its very best*, a place where the herd celebrates this in us because it understands that what is truly good for each and every one of us will ultimately be good for all of us.

A GUT CHECK

It's an enormous paradigm leap to go from relying on what is outside of you to tell you what to
do or how to be, to checking in with yourself
first. It's so much easier to check out of our inner
knowing as we get swept up in the daily
demands and the overwhelm of all the choices
we navigate each day, especially when we're
immersed in a sea of opinions about how to do
it all.

But if we are to feel empowered in our own
bodies in the presence of others, while coming
from a place of balance and wholeness, we must
commit to a regular space and time we can
count on to get in touch with what we know and
feel to be true. A place where you can hear
yourself without apologizing, toning down, or
justifying what you're experiencing. A place
where you can practice on your own so that
when you are with the group, you have a solid
and centered reference point for what you need
and what you value.

What would it be like to carve out and commit to a regular time and space to show up, exactly as you are, in order to do *a gut check*? It doesn't have to be a long time, and it doesn't have to look like anything other than you being on your own. A regular time that gives you access to your thoughts and feelings, along with an inner sensing of what is happening in your life. A space that allows you to welcome all of who you are.

Of course, there will be thoughts that will come in attached to other people and what you imagine they believe, think and need from you. Let yourself notice those thought patterns, and let it be. You might even say to yourself, *I know what they think, but this space is about checking in with what I think.*

In this space, you do not need to have any answers. As a matter of fact, getting in touch with yourself in this way will generate *a ton* of questions. This is normal and to be expected. Questions will let you know you are on the right track. For at the very heart of this time on your own is about you developing greater self-trust in the face of a world demanding you listen to everyone else.

Maybe your gut check is in the shower, or waiting in line. Maybe it is lying in bed before falling asleep or upon awakening. Maybe it is a walk, meditation or a yoga class. The externals of the space do not matter. What matters is that *daily* you check in with yourself. *Daily* you notice whether or not what you are pondering leaves you with a settled feeling in your gut or a queasy, uneasy, tense, tight, you name it, feeling.

That feeling in your gut is your answer. Whether you can name why this is so, or not. Whether you can prove it or not. Put 'them' and what 'they think' aside. *What does your gut say?* This is a powerful and honest predictor of what is happening for you in the presence of others. The socially conditioned mind will not initially be the one to tell you something is not working when it comes to the herd. *But your body will.*

Give lots and lots of space to any questions, confusions, frustrations or disappointments around your life with others. Get in the regular habit of questioning whether or not you must squelch your real and necessary instincts for the 'good of the whole.' *What does that even mean?* Do we only have one choice in this regard? Is it true that going along with a sick herd is actually good for the whole?

These are lifelong, complex and earth-shattering questions to pose. But for us to even have the courage to question at this level, to even begin to think for ourselves in this way, requires a mindset that says, *When I am better, we are all better.* The converse is also true: *A healthy herd would never, ever, ask, expect or demand that you choose between belonging and doing right by your own body.* This one statement alone can serve as your True North when navigating the waters of belonging and self-care.

A Vision

Finally, what if you decided to act on your own truth in the company of others, no matter how difficult, awkward, inconvenient or socially inappropriate it might seem? And what if doing so is ultimately the best thing for all concerned, despite any difficulties or hesitations you might have? Despite whether or not it's easy to do, say or hear.

It takes clarity, conviction and courage
to stand in the truth of your experience when
it differs from those around you.

But the rewards are great for both you and everyone you meet. *Can you imagine what could happen if we all took responsibility for our own experience while in the presence of another, and acted on that as thoughtfully and straightforwardly as we could? Could you imagine letting go of the social niceties that keep you pinned to the wrong things? Can you imagine how good it would feel to not have to fake your way through an interaction or dumb yourself down to make others feel better?*

What would it be like for you to belong, exactly as you are? Maybe you're thinking there is no way this is possible. Is it a strenuous choice? *It is.* Will it take practice and negotiation? *Definitely.* Will we need lots and lots of us to have a conversation around deciding what is best for us and still belong? *Yes.*

Let's remember though the time when everyone believed the world was flat, and a growing number of visionaries insisted the world was round. What if we could take this same leap together and move beyond the fears, hesitations and doubts to hold a new truth that said, *Caring for ourselves is caring for others.* Even when it means breaking from ingrained, outdated, and even sick, herd behaviors.

There are lots of unanswered and unspoken questions here. Ones that only each one of us can choose to take up and explore. For it will only be by challenging the outdated stories we tell ourselves around who we are and what we must do to belong that we will ever be able to discover what is truly possible for all of us when we choose to care for ourselves as the basis for healthy belonging.

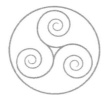

The End of This Journey

*"We shall not cease from exploration, and the end
of all our exploring will be to arrive where we started
and know the place for the first time."*

- T.S. Eliot

Wow. Here we are at the end of this portion of The Embodied Journey. We have traveled far together, and my prayer for you is that you continue stepping forward each day in learning to care for your precious body. How you think about your body and your life in it, sets the course for how you will live in the world. How you treat yourself is not separate from how you treat others, the Earth or how it is that you feel about being alive.

This is a big deal. I would say the biggest ever because we are really talking about how you will live this one life of yours. What you will believe in. Where you will put your efforts. What it is that you will reach for, *and what it is that you will not tolerate.*

I wish you many blessings on your continued journey. May you go on to share whatever you discover with those around you. May you realize your truest Nature and may you see that this body of yours, the very one that allows you to be here, is a portal into something vast, mysterious and so worth getting to know. Thank you for being here and for taking the time to care for yourself. May this ending become a new beginning.

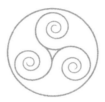

Acknowledgments

To Leah who came into my life at exactly the right time with your natural and no-nonsense approach to birthing a creation. You're a great midwife.

To Sara, Steph, Tracey and Vici who have been an incredible circle of support. You women have held and encouraged me, each in your own way, to be brave enough to do something like this.

To Joanna, you are a soul sister to me and you are the reason this book took the form it did, along with the reason why so many other blessings have come my way. May we both realize...

To Maddie and Jack, I love you both. My life took its true shape when you came into the world. May you be so blessed.

And to Steve, my soulmate and partner in creating a more beautiful world. You saw me long before I did, and you have kept the faith for me when I could not. You have mended my broken heart more times than I can count. Please stay for as long as you can.

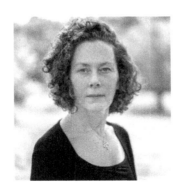

About the Author

Susan McNamara, M.A., CHHC is the founder of *The Healer Within*, an online health and healing community for women. She also writes the weekly blog, *Medicine for the People*. For more than 30 years she has been exploring, teaching and most of all, living what it means to be in a body in a trusting, sacred and nourishing way.

In addition to her Masters in Counseling Psychology, as well as being trained and educated at the Doctoral Level in Clinical Psychology, Susan is a Certified Holistic Health Counselor, Professional-Level Kripalu Yoga Teacher, Journeydance Guide and Shamanic Practitioner.

www.RememberingWhatMattersMost.com

Made in the USA
Middletown, DE
18 July 2022